Abdominal Strength for Life® 2

Advanced Exercises for
Leaner and Stronger Core Muscles
After 40, 60, &!

Josef Arnould, D.C.

Abdominal Strength for Life® 2

Advanced Exercises for Leaner and Stronger Core Muscles After 40, 60, &!

© 2020 Josef Arnould, D.C.

Published in Easthampton, Massachusetts by Strength for Life® Health & Fitness Center. Strength for Life® is a registered U.S. Trademark of CX Associates of Northampton, Inc. www.StrengthForLife.com

ISBN 978-0-9989617-5-0

Photographs by Caitlin Arnould, Alan Robinson, and Sarah Whiteley

Disclaimer

An essential principle set forth in this book is that, prior to making any changes in his or her exercise or dietary habits, each reader is personally responsible to communicate directly and in person with at least one healthcare professional who is knowledgeable and experienced in the fields of exercise healthcare and nutritional science. The present work advances general guidelines for exercising and eating healthfully. It does not present an exercise prescription for any one specific person. The author assumes no responsibility or liability for such personal use. All readers who intend to use the information presented in this book are urged to discuss their exercise and dietary plans with their personal physician(s), especially with doctors who themselves exercise regularly and intelligently.

Dedication

As many of you, in late March of 2020 I was infected by the virulent virus that has taken and continues to take the lives of so many people throughout the world. I had the good fortune to be attended by my loving wife Abby almost 24/7 during ten days of delirium and roller-coaster fevers. Just as I was emerging from this battle, I developed swelling, redness, heat, and pain in my left ankle, which turned out to be blood clots in the superficial veins in that region. Hence, I needed another week of intensive nursing care, which she provided with patience and tenderness. Therefore, this book is dedicated first to my wife, Abby Arnould.

Second, I dedicate this work to my children, Caitlin, Dylan, Meghan, and Holly, who sent daily bouquets of love and encouragement that helped me stay positive throughout the darkness of this ordeal. Along with them, I dedicate this work to my brothers and sisters, as well as to my niece Brianna Beaumont, RN, and her partner, Clayton Wheatley, MD, for their vigilant medical observations and advice from afar, to Peter Morse, MD, who diagnosed the blood clots in my ankle, and to Jonathan Marsh, MD, who guided me through follow-up treatment for those clots.

Third, I dedicate this work to my star student and friend, Ted Davidson, who ran errands almost daily to keep our household supplied with food and other necessities. He also shuttled me twice to and from the emergency room of our local hospital.

Next, I dedicate this work to all the medical staff persons, first responders, nursing home workers, public service professionals and others who have done everything they possibly could, often at great risk to their own health, to help their fellow citizens get through this enormously challenging health crisis.

Finally, I dedicate this book to many governors, both Republican and Democratic, who took command during this crisis by implementing public health measures that were crucial to preventing this virus from overwhelming us completely. Their decisive and clearly articulated actions, based upon the best scientific and medical information available at that time, guided us through uncharted dark waters, saving the lives of thousands of people in their states and in this country. This is the brand of honest and intelligent leadership we need on the national and international levels now, and in coming decades, to confront new epidemics and other global crises that do and will threaten the habitability of our planet for human life. Therefore, although the first purpose of this book is to improve our own physical fitness and personal health, may it also lead us to a higher dedication. Let us pledge now to work for improving the fitness of our environment and , thus, to achieve better health for all living creatures on planet Earth in the future.

Table of Contents

Introduction

My name is Josef Arnould. I am the 72-year-old director of a chiropractic and exercise healthcare clinic in Easthampton, Massachusetts, U.S.A. I have been fortunate to have had the opportunity to devote my entire professional career to teaching individuals how, by exercising intelligently, they can realize their individual potentials for excellent health and amazing physical capabilities. By "excellent health" and "amazing physical capabilities," I mean the capacities to perform with elegance and excellence the required and desired physical activities of our daily lives. This includes not only clothing, feeding, and bathing ourselves, but also, being able to walk, garden, dance, play tennis and perform hundreds of other physical activities we enjoy doing. Stated another way, my job has been and remains to inspire every person I encounter to strive for the freedom of vibrant physical health. In the 1990s, to summarize this quest, I coined and trademarked the phrase "Strength for Life®," a term which I request you allow me to define below.

First, "strength," in terms of physical health, is not merely the ability to move or lift heavy objects. Rather, it is an essential quality of human health. It is the force we use to move our bodies gracefully and powerfully in completing everyday tasks <u>and</u> in performing a myriad of other physical activities that engender meaning and excitement in our minds and hearts. "Strength" is an attribute of health that must be cultivated every day. When we nurture our bodies by exercising intelligently, we maximize our potential for lifelong strength. Conversely, if we fail to stimulate our bodies with challenging exercise every day, we lose our strength prematurely and surrender the opportunity to enjoy the independence of good health for as long in life as possible.

Secondly, the final two words of this phrase, "for life," suggest multiple meanings. Overtly, these words proclaim we should develop and maintain the quality of strength for the entire duration of our lives. Just as importantly, however, "for life" means we should endeavor also to savor the body-wide shivers of excitement we feel when we are physically active. I call this feeling "the thrill of exertion."

No matter what your age, if you accept the challenge of the advanced exercises in this book, welcome to a world where we nurture our strength and yearn for the thrilling experience of being physically active every day.

Josef Arnould, D.C.

Two other books in the Strength for Life® Series by Josef Arnould, D.C

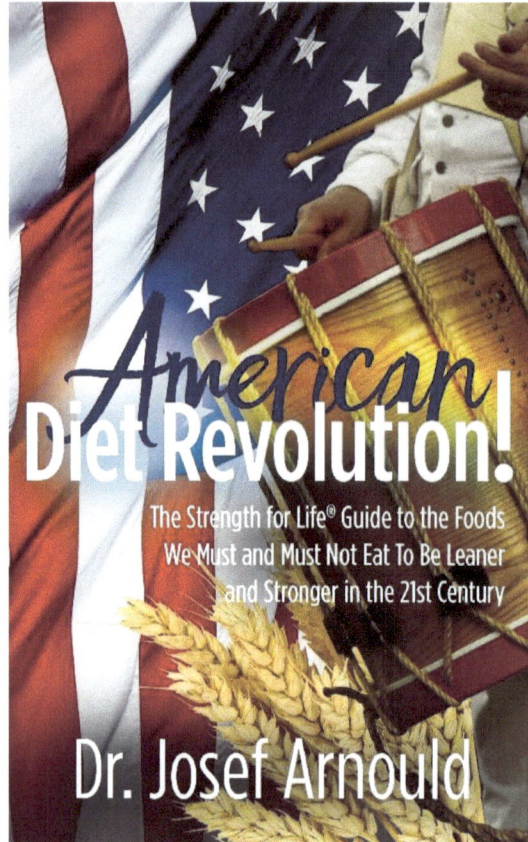

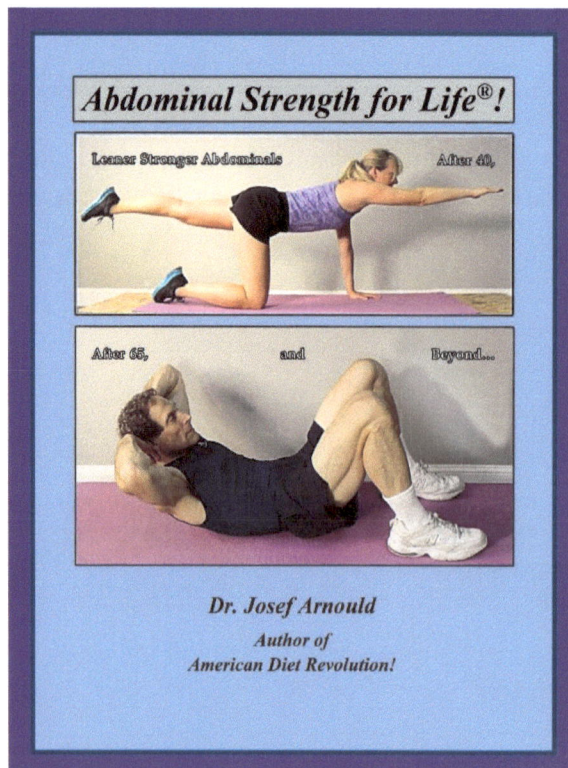

Chapter One

Introducing Abdominal Strength for Life® 2

As its subtitle proclaims, this book presents advanced level exercises for the development of compact strength in the core muscles of the human body. To perform advanced exercises safely and effectively, we must master first the foundational exercises which precede them. Therefore, before we commence with the first series of advanced core exercises in Chapter Two, it is important to reach a common understanding of at least five essential points regarding core exercises. If you do not attain this level of understanding, it is my contention you will jeopardize your chances for success with advanced level exercises and increase your risk for injury as you attempt to perform them.

Point One

These are advanced core exercises. They are more challenging versions of the fundamental core exercises presented as the beginning level of training in *Abdominal Strength for Life®! (AbSfL*, Volume 1). If you have not yet mastered these exercises, you must begin doing so now. Virtually all advanced level core exercises are simply more demanding versions of beginning level exercises. These foundational exercises may seem simple at first. However, the more precisely and intensively you perform them, the more precisely and intensively you will be able to perform advanced level core exercises. Personally, one or two days per week these foundational exercises are the only core exercises I perform. And even today, after doing them for more than forty years, I still feel I am improving in how well I do these fundamental exercises and how much benefit I derive from them.

For free, you can access a video presentation of the foundational core exercises of the Strength for Life® program by visiting www.StrengthForLife.com, clicking "Videos," then "videocasts," and selecting "Episode 1: Core Exercises." If you desire a deeper understanding of these fundamental exercises, at the same website you can order either the economical ebook version of *Abdominal Strength for Life®!* Volume One or the beautiful, 135-page print version. The print version is a great value because you will refer to it frequently for many years.

I would like to emphasize especially that, before you tackle the advanced core exercises in this book, you study and practice two foundational exercises which are crucial for your success and safety: the Abdominal Vacuum and the Lower Abdominal Curl. Perfecting the vacuum is essential for building a compact muscular core. Even more importantly, by perfecting the Lower Abdominal Curl, you protect the integrity of your lower spinal complex. In the first volume of the *AbSfL* series, these are taught as separate and distinct exercises. However, at the advanced level of the present volume, these are not performed as separate exercises, but instead, as intrinsic elements of virtually every advanced exercise.

Point Two

Abdominal muscles and core muscles are not synonymous terms. Our "core" consists of much more than just the "abs." Yes, the abdominals are front and center, the rock stars of an ensemble we call the core. But they are not soloists. They are surrounded by and supported by several other bands of muscles that encircle the middle third of the human body. In nearly every human activity, and in almost all "core" exercises, these highly interrelated muscle groups work in concert, not in isolation.

In *AbSfL* Volume 1, I define the core muscles of the human body as the "lower torso/hip complex," i.e. the entire circumference of skeletal muscles attached from the bottom of the ribcage to the tops of the knees. However, in *AbSfL*, Volume 2, you will discover quickly that my definition of "core muscles" has been expanded even further. In advanced training, our "core" includes muscles of the hips, shoulders, and neck as they attach to the trunk of the human body. Why this expansion? The answer is straightforward. Functionally, i.e., as we engage ourselves in more challenging and complex physical movements, we call upon more muscle groups to participate. The band becomes an orchestra. Therefore, I have expanded the definition of our core to include all muscle groups of the limbs and the neck that attach to our torsos. For instance, in several advanced core exercises in this book, you will feel coordinated muscle movements in and development of flexible strength in the rotator cuff muscles of your shoulders. As you develop a heightened awareness of the increasing functional integrity of these peripheral core muscles, you will feel how intimately they interact in coordination with movements of your chest, back, and even your abdominal muscles. Likewise, as flexible strength of your neck muscles improves, you will feel how important these muscles are to successful execution of many abdominal exercises. When you reach this stage personal psychomotor awareness, you have transcended the ridiculous misconception that your core muscles are only "six-pack abs."

Point Three

Achieving a leaner midsection is not primarily the result of your exercise regimen. The qualities of the foods and beverages we choose to eat and drink are the most important factors in attaining and maintaining a healthy level of bodyfat. Doing hours of core muscle exercises every day will not compensate for eating and drinking foods and beverages which cause us to store fat and which inflame the organ systems of our bodies. In 2019, Morgan James Publishing released my dynamic book on nutrition and weight loss, *American Diet Revolution!* At www.StrengthForLife.com you will find links to purchase either the print or ebook version of this work at very modest prices.

Point Four

Just doing an exercise is not enough. By this negative statement I am asking you to transcend the mechanical way of exercising, that is, rattling off a very high number of rapid repetitions and stopping when you reach that arbitrary number. Instead of counting off repetitions, I ask you to concentrate intently upon the sensations you are experiencing in your body as you alternately contract and then lengthen the target muscles in each exercise. Put another way, for maximal strength and health value, what you are thinking about and what you are feeling as you perform an exercise are at least as important as the physical movements occurring in your body.

Developmental exercises (physical training that builds muscle mass, strength, flexibility, coordination, agility, etc.) are not merely mechanistic activities. Each exercise should become an intensely personal and immediate psychomotor experience, a lively dialogue between your brain and whatever elements of your body are being challenged in that specific exercise.

Point Five

More Is Not Better; Better is Better. Most core muscle exercises do not require the use of heavy forms of resistance, such as heavy dumbbells, kettlebells, or heavy medicine balls. Instead of using heavy resistances, many exercisers resort to doing dozens or even hundreds of repetitions in rapid-fire succession. Their hypothesis is that doing a high number of repetitions will compensate for the lack of heavy resistances and, thus, build more strength and leanness in their core muscles. In actual performance, however, as they rattle off oodles of mind-numbing repetitions, their minds wander far away from feeling the movements in the target muscles of their bodies. People who train in this manner not only waste time and energy; in most cases, they almost certainly do not achieve the results to which they aspire. Just as importantly, they deprive themselves of the marvelous brain-body experience we enjoy when we concentrate intently on what we are feeling, as opposed to merely counting how many repetitions we are doing.

After more than 35 years of teaching adults from ages 16 to 95, I state unequivocally that the biggest mistake most people make in performing core exercises is doing high numbers of repetitions very fast, through limited ranges of motion, and with quick herky-jerky movements. On the other hand, if we savor the sensations in our bodies as we perform a limited number of repetitions slowly, through a full range of potential movement for each target muscle group, we learn to communicate intimately with ourselves as we experience the thrill of intensive physical exertion. In this context, exercise is not painful: it becomes exciting!

Based upon the five points presented in the paragraphs above, on the following page I present *Fundamentals of Strength for Life® Core Exercise Performance*, which are guidelines for performing all the exercises in this book effectively and enjoyably. I promise that you will find many of these exercises to be unique. More importantly, however, I promise that the way in which you learn to do these exercises will be even more unique. You will learn to move your body in ways you never thought possible, even when you were younger than you are today. What is more, your newly developed awareness of your physical capabilities will inspire you to undertake new activities, activities you never felt bold enough or energetic enough to attempt previously. When you reach this stage, you will know you have taken training exercises and infused them deeply into every other physical aspect of your life. There is great joy to be discovered in developing our Strength for Life®!

Fundamentals of Strength for Life® Core Exercise Performance

1. **Every repetition of every core exercise has two distinct phases.**
   a. Contraction Phase. From a fully stretched Beginning Position, contract your target muscles slowly as you initiate movement toward an intensely contracted Peak Position. Pause momentarily.
   b. Extension Phase. From the fully contracted Peak Position, return slowly to a fully stretched Beginning Position. Pause briefly,

2. **Pause momentarily at the end of each phase**.
   Pausing as you reach the end of each phase provides a moment to focus intently upon contracting or lengthening your target muscles in the upcoming phase. In addition, at the beginning of the Contraction Phase, if you must initiate movement from a complete standstill, you will build more flexible strength in your target muscles than if you were to simply bounce from the previous repetition without a pause. Ten repetitions performed with a pause at the end of each phase of every repetition will create more flexible strength in your target muscles than a hundred done with bouncing and herky-jerky haste.

3. **Concentrate intently as you contract and lengthen your target muscles through every inch of movement of every repetition**.
   It is not enough to just do an exercise. Strive always to feel what is happening in your target muscles as you perform that exercise.

4. **The breathing pattern for every exercise is: Exhale throughout the Contraction Phase; Inhale throughout the Extension Phase.**
   a. In the Beginning Position, before you begin movement, inhale.
   b. Begin exhaling as soon as you initiate movement in the Contraction Phase. By exhaling as you compress the abdominal and thoracic cavities, you reduce the risk of a Valsalva Maneuver, which can impede the flow of blood and oxygen to the heart. Continue exhaling until you reach the Peak Position, where you will pause.
   c. As you initiate the Extension Phase, begin to inhale. Continue to inhale slowly and deeply until you reach the Beginning Position.
   d. When you breathe in this pattern, the rate of your bodily movements becomes synchronous with your rate of deep, slow breathing. Slow, steady, graceful movement is ideal for developing strength throughout the entire ranges of motion of your core muscles.

Chapter Two

Advanced Abdominal Medley #1

As we begin the first of the three advanced core muscle workouts presented in this book, there are four additional concepts we should consider. Being aware of these concepts as we train will maximize the benefits we derive from the investments of time, money, and energy that performance of these exercises requires.

1. Each of the three advanced level core muscle workouts presented in this volume are organized as a "medley," meaning the individual exercises are to be performed as a continuous sequence with a minimum of rest between each exercise. As advanced trainees, we are always striving to improve our aerobic fitness and muscular stamina. Moving promptly from exercise to exercise in each medley, with almost no rest between these exercises, will elevate your heart rate to a modest training level for the 15 to 20 minutes required to complete each medley.

2. In the photos of many exercises, you will note my hands are placed in a reversed position, i.e., with the back of my fingers against the back of my neck. As explained in Volume 1, this positioning allows for some neck support but prevents a trainee from pulling too forcefully on his or her neck and head.

3. You cannot perform safely several of the advanced exercises in this book if you have weak neck muscles. As you attempt many of these challenging exercises, you will feel considerable demands for flexible strength in your neck. Volume 1 contains a separate chapter devoted only to neck exercises that you can and should do regularly.

4. Finally, a friendly reminder. What you are thinking about and what you are feeling as you perform each repetition of each exercise are vastly more important than how many repetitions you do. I call this "internalizing your exercise experience." It is the exact opposite of rattling off dozens of rapid-fire repetitions. When you learn to exercise with an ongoing deep awareness of what you are feeling, you are truly on the way to the advanced level of physical training.

Advanced SfL Abdominal Medley #1

1. Agility Ball Lower Ab Curl/Vacuum & Leg Press to Full Spine Extension
  a. Primary Target Muscle Group: Lower Rectus Abdominis
  b. Secondary Target Muscle Groups: Upper Rectus & Transverse Abdominis. This exercise reinforces excellent upper spinal posture, an essential component of vibrant health. However, if your neck muscles are weak, you must place your hands behind your neck instead of on your hips.
  c. Directions
      (1) Position yourself with your lower back against the side of an agility ball, hands on your hips, your knees bent, feet flat, and glutes close to the floor. Allow your head and neck to extend backward to a degree that feels comfortable.
      (2) Push your lower back into the ball. In this deep squat position, do an abdominal vacuum (**Top photo**). This is the Beginning Position.
      (3) As you start to exhale, do a strong lower abdominal curl into the ball and begin a leg press. During your ascent, keep your head and neck in extension, which will remind you why we all need to do neck strengthening exercises. Continue to push your lower back forcefully into the ball. To intensify the contractions in your lower rectus abdominis even more, imagine someone is punching you with a fist just below the umbilicus (**Middle**).
      (4) As you complete a leg press to full knee extension, allow your head and neck to extend backward and downward as far as your brain tells you is safe. Pause momentarily in this Peak Position to savor both the powerful contractions in your entire rectus abdominis and the restful sensation of being in a supported position of full spine extension (**Bottom photo**).
      (5) Inhale as you descend to the beginning position; do another abdominal vacuum; continue using your lower rectus abdominis to press into the ball; and maintain your head and neck in extension.
      (6) Pause when you reach the beginning position, then repeat steps (3) through (5) 10 to 15 times. Perform each repetition slowly so you can feel the complex sequence of muscles challenged by this exercise.

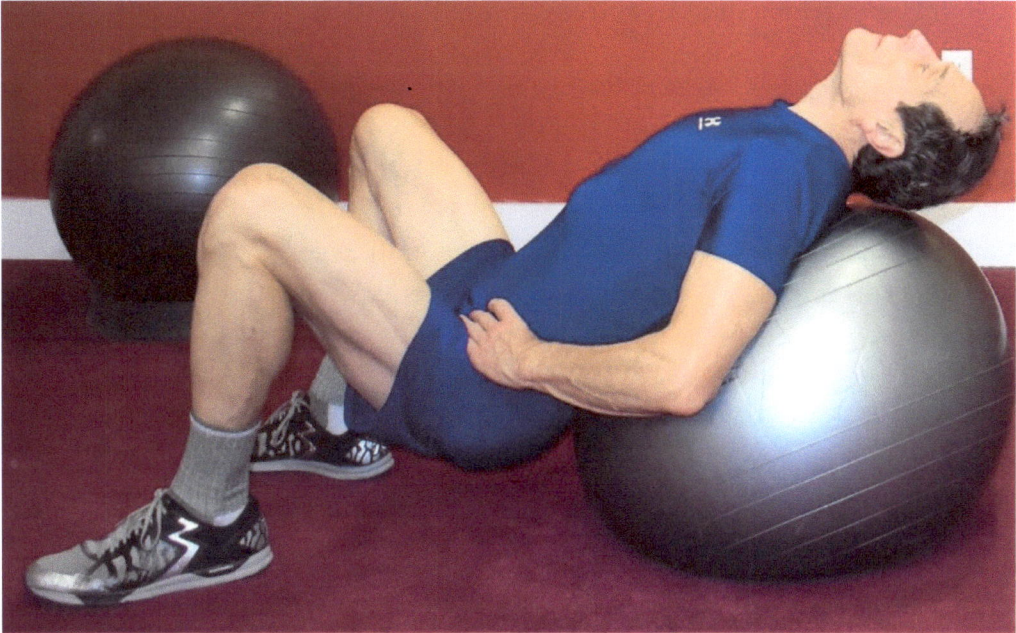
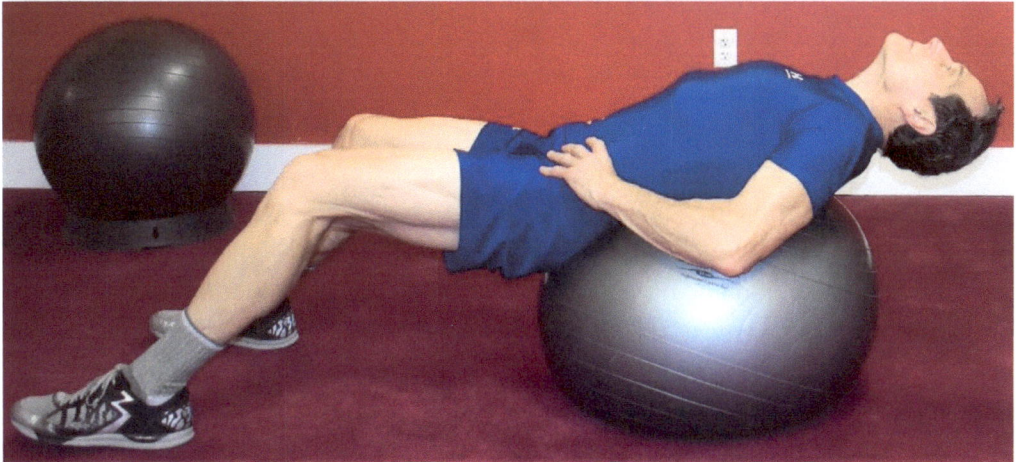
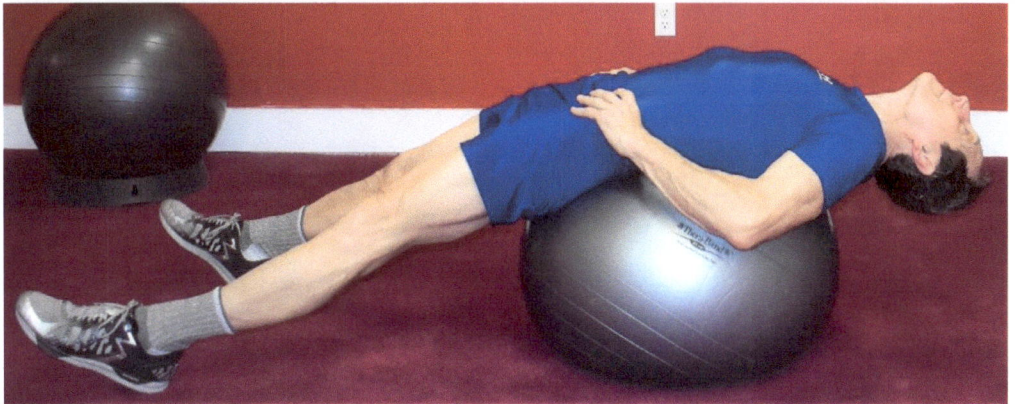

2. Agility Ball Upper Abdominal Curl from Spinal Extension

a. Primary Target Muscle Group: Upper Rectus Abdominis
Secondary Target Muscles: Lower Rectus, Transverse Abdominis.

b. Two unique elements of this version of the upper abdominal curl are (1) that you strive for full spinal extension in the beginning position and (2) that in peak contraction position your chest, shoulders and neck are only parallel with the floor. In other words, this exercise ends where most abdominal curl exercises begin. Thus, we are we are building flexible core muscle strength in a range of motion most other exercises ignore entirely.

c. Directions

(1) Lie supine on the ball, your torso parallel to the floor, your feet wide apart, your knees bent at right angles, your lower sternum above the center of the ball, your hands reversed and supporting your neck.

(2) Allow your head and shoulders to extend backward and downward until you feel a full stretch in your abdominals, the Beginning Position (**Top**). Seeing the wall behind you, do an abdominal vacuum. Inhale.

(3) As you begin to exhale, slowly perform first a strong lower abdominal curl into the ball to initiate upward movement of your head and shoulders (**Middle**), followed immediately but smoothly by slow, controlled curling movements in your upper abdominals until your torso reaches the Peak Position, which is approximately parallel to the floor (**Bottom**). Pause briefly to savor this sensation.

(4) Inhale deeply as you lower your torso, shoulders, and head slowly backward and downward to the beginning position, uncurling your abdominal muscles in the reverse order of your ascent and performing another abdominal vacuum on your way down. Pause momentarily before repeating steps (3) and (4).

(5) With as much concentration as you can muster, enjoy 10-15 slow repetitions of this invigorating exercise.

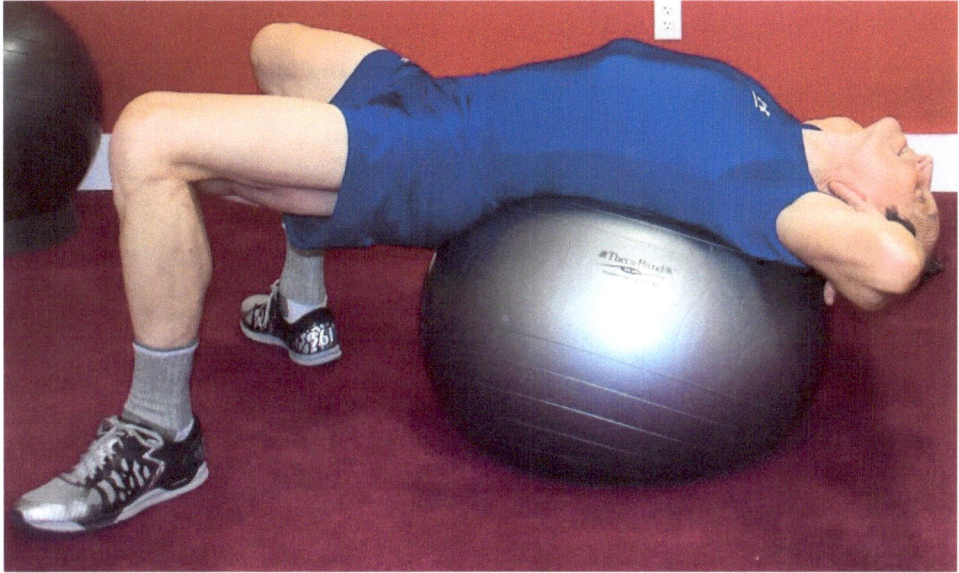
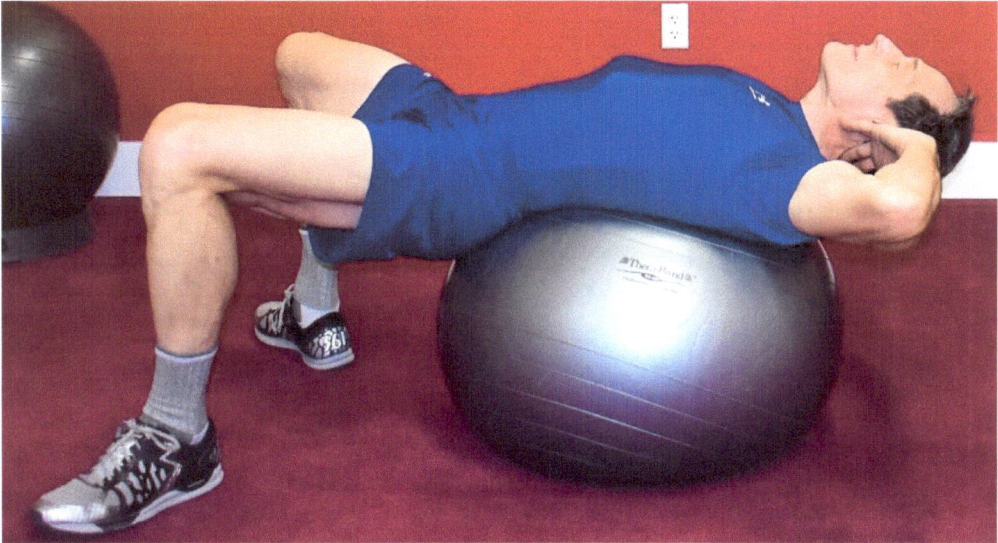
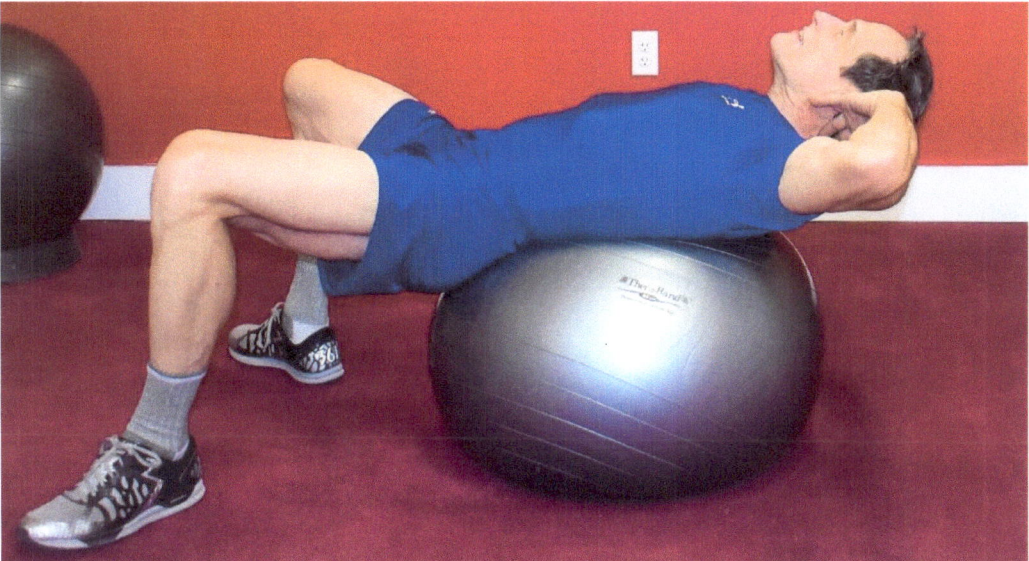

3. Agility Ball Diagonal Abdominal Curl/ Elbow Pointing Overhead

a. Primary Target Muscles: External Obliques, Upper/Lower Rectus Abdominis, Transverse Abdominis

b. In performing the Agility Ball Diagonal Curl in *Abdominal Strength for Life® !*, we pointed the elbow toward the opposite knee as we curled upward, forward and diagonally Although that is a challenging intermediate level exercise for the rotational muscles of the lower torso/hip complex, it is easy in comparison to this version. Here, we point the elbow toward a point on the ceiling directly overhead, which increases the thrill of exertion.

c. Direction

(1) Lie on your back over the center of the ball. Place your left hand behind your neck. For balance, place the fingers of your right hand on the floor next to the ball. Turning your head to the left, allow your left shoulder and elbow to descend toward the floor, until you can feel a great stretch in the muscles on that side of your ribcage. Perform an abdominal vacuum and inhale. This is the Beginning Position (**Top**).

(2) As you begin to exhale, initiate upward movement by performing a lower abdominal curl, followed immediately by a rotating upper abdominal curl in which you raise and turn your head, left shoulder, and elbow upward and to the right. As you turn, pick out a spot on the ceiling directly overhead and begin moving your elbow toward it (**Middle**).

(3) Continue to raise and rotate your torso until your left elbow is pointing directly at the spot overhead (**Bottom**). Your target muscles feel magnificently contracted. Pause momentarily to enjoy this Peak Position.

(4) Inhale deeply and slowly as you uncurl your left elbow, head, and shoulder back to the beginning position. As you unwind, use your lower rectus to keep your lower back pressed firmly into the ball and do another abdominal vacuum.

(5) Perform 10 repetitions on the left, then 10 on the right.

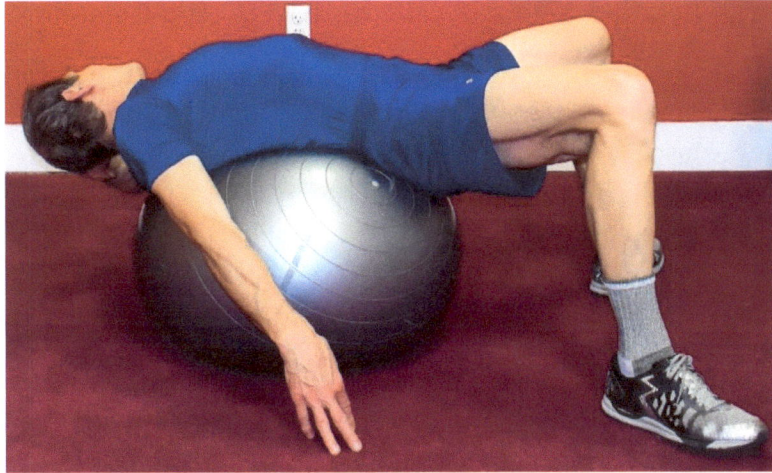
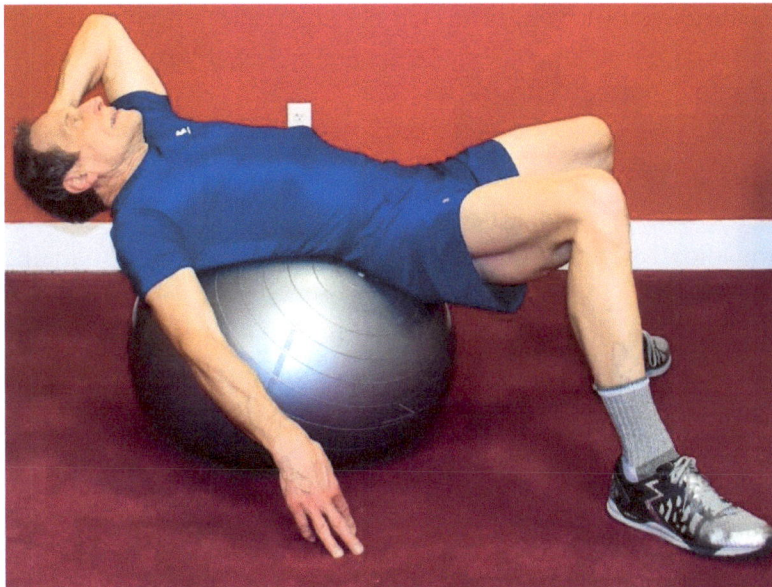
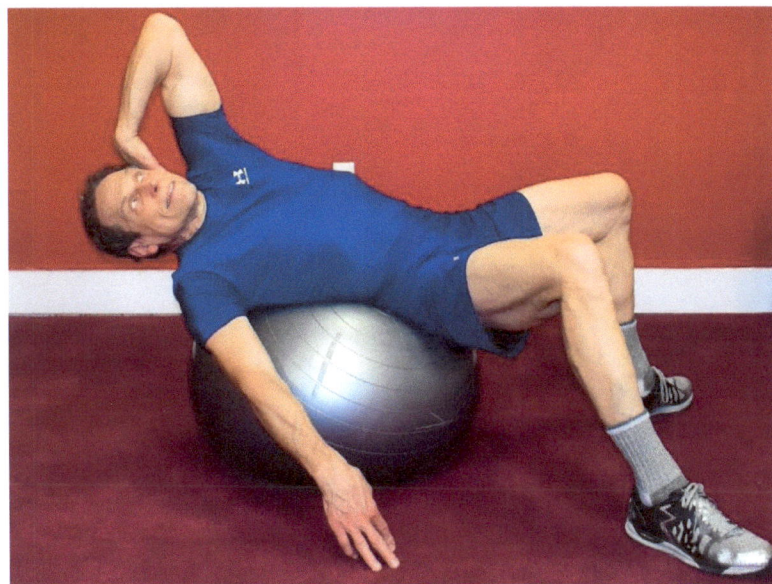

4. Agility Ball, Reversely Rotating, Side Jackknife w/ External Hip Rotation

a. Primary Target Muscles: External Rotators and Abductors of the Hip; Quadratus Lumborum; Serratus Posterior; Latissimus Dorsi; Trapezius; Supraspinatus, Infraspinatus; Posterior Deltoids Secondary Target Muscles: Transverse Abdominis, Cervical Rotators

b. Our goal here is to develop flexible strength and coordination in all interrelated muscle groups of the Lower Torso/Hip Complex, Upper Torso and Shoulders, and the neck.

c. Directions

(1) Lie on your right side on an agility ball, the tip of your lower sternum approximately over the center of the ball. Move your right foot 12 inches forward, your left foot 12 inches backward, and put your reversed left hand behind your neck. Lower your head, left shoulder, and left elbow toward the floor as you turn your torso rightward and downward to the Beginning Position (**Top**). Inhale and perform an abdominal vacuum.

(2) Begin to exhale as you lift your head, left shoulder, and left elbow while turning your torso backward and upward. Simultaneously, abduct and externally rotate your left leg and turn your left big toe toward the ceiling (**Middle**).

(3) Continue to raise and externally rotate your head, left shoulder, elbow, leg, and big toe upward and backward until both your elbow and your toe point toward the ceiling, the Peak Position (**Bottom**). Pause momentarily.

(4) Inhale as you allow all moving members of your body to return to their respective beginning positions and, of course, enjoy an abdominal vacuum as you descend.

(5) Repeat Steps (2) – (4) for a total of 10 repetitions, then.

(6) Perform 10 exciting repetitions while lying on your left side.

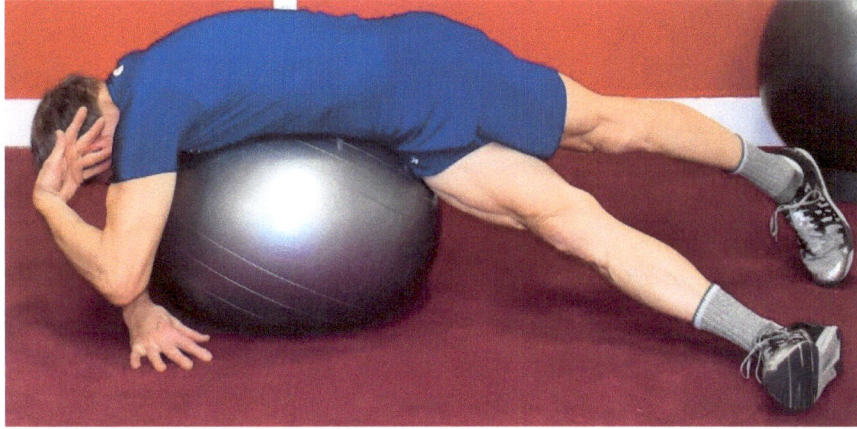

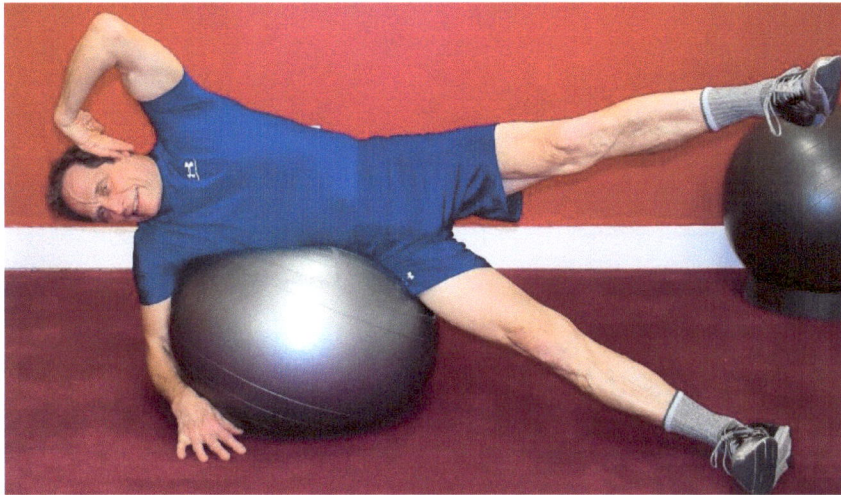

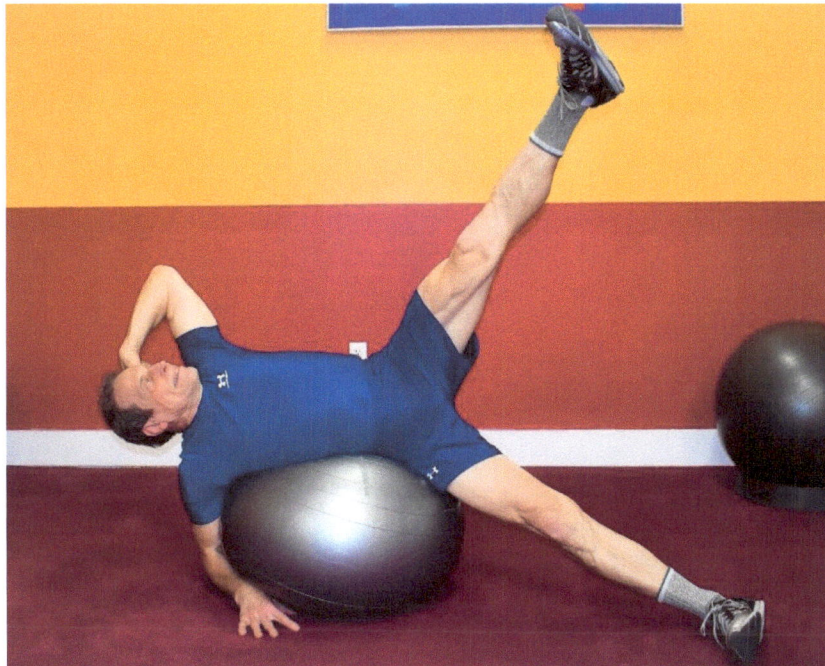

5. Agility Ball Pointer Head to Toe

a. Primary Target Muscles: Erector Spinae, Hip Extensors and Flexors Secondary Target Muscles: Flexors and Extensors of the Knee, Dorsiflexors and Plantar Flexors of the Ankle and Foot, Transverse Abdominis, Neck extensors

b. This exercise typifies how we can use our core muscles to cultivate flexible strength and coordination, physical attributes critical to achieving and maintaining the freedom of whole-body health as we age.

c. Directions

(1) Lie face down on an agility ball with the lower tip of your sternum approximately over the center of the ball. Place your hands on the floor in front, straighten your legs until you feel a stretch in your hamstrings, and stretch the tendons on the bottom of your feet and toes against the floor behind. This is the Beginning Position (**Top**).

(2) As you begin to inhale, draw your right elbow backward and your left knee forward to sides of the ball. At the same time, do an abdominal vacuum and let your head move downward until your chin nearly touches the ball (**Middle**). Pause momentarily.

(3) As you begin to exhale: lift your head to look straight ahead; raise your right arm and point forward with your fingers; move your left foot backward until the knee is straight and your toes are pointing behind you. This is the Peak Position (**Bottom**). In addition to mild contractions up and down the length of your spine and in your right shoulder muscles, you should feel a stretch in the muscles on the top of your left foot and in your left hamstrings. Pause momentarily to savor these sensations. This is the difference between really feeling your target muscles, as opposed to doing an exercise mechanically.

(4) Inhale and do an abdominal vacuum as you return to the beginning position. Pause momentarily, then perform steps **(2)-(3)** on the opposite side. Inhale as your left elbow goes back and the right knee forward; exhale as you point ahead with your left hand and behind with your right toes.

(5) Continue alternating. Enjoy 10-15 repetitions on each side.

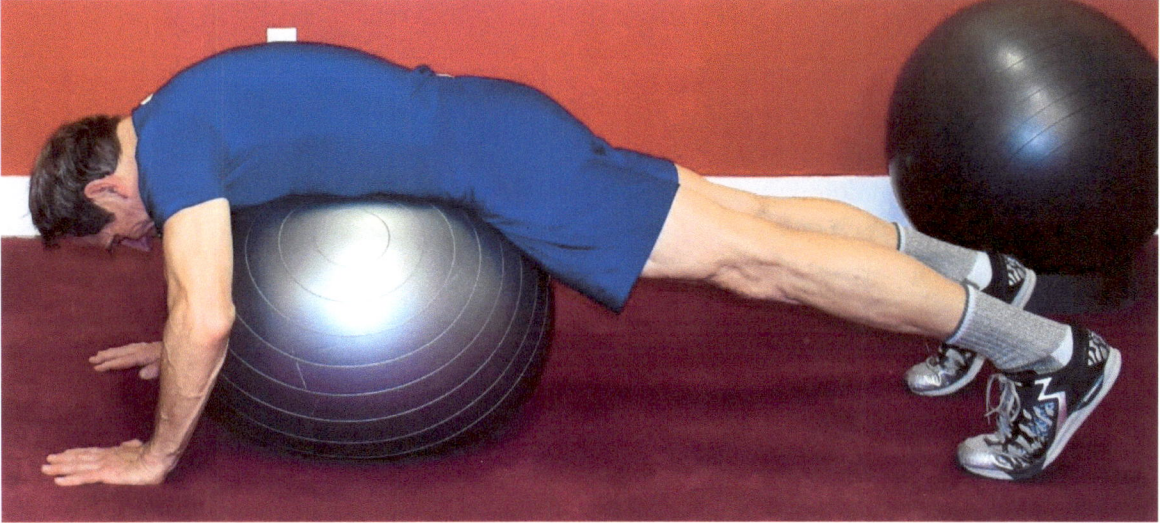
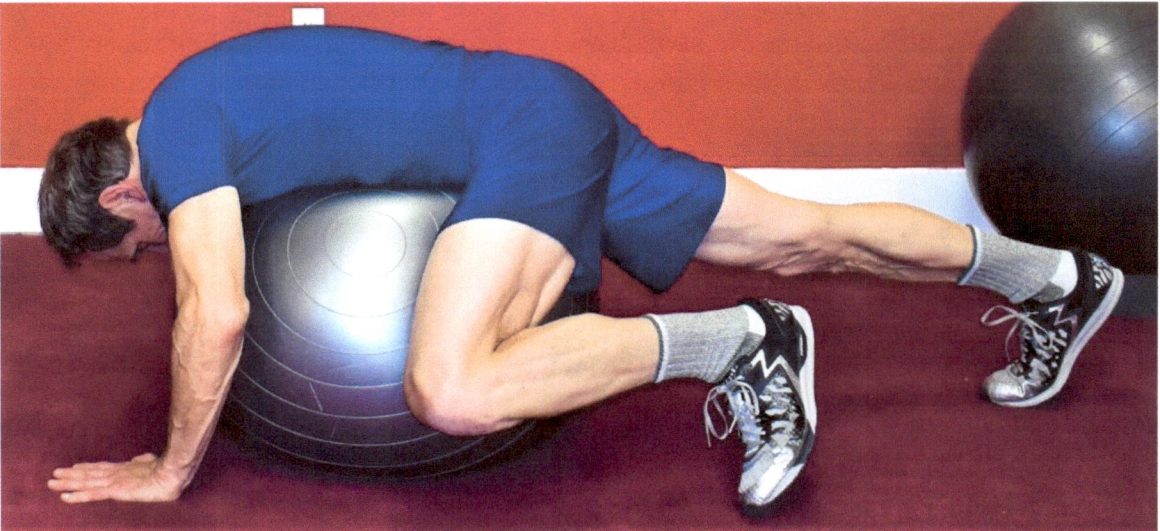
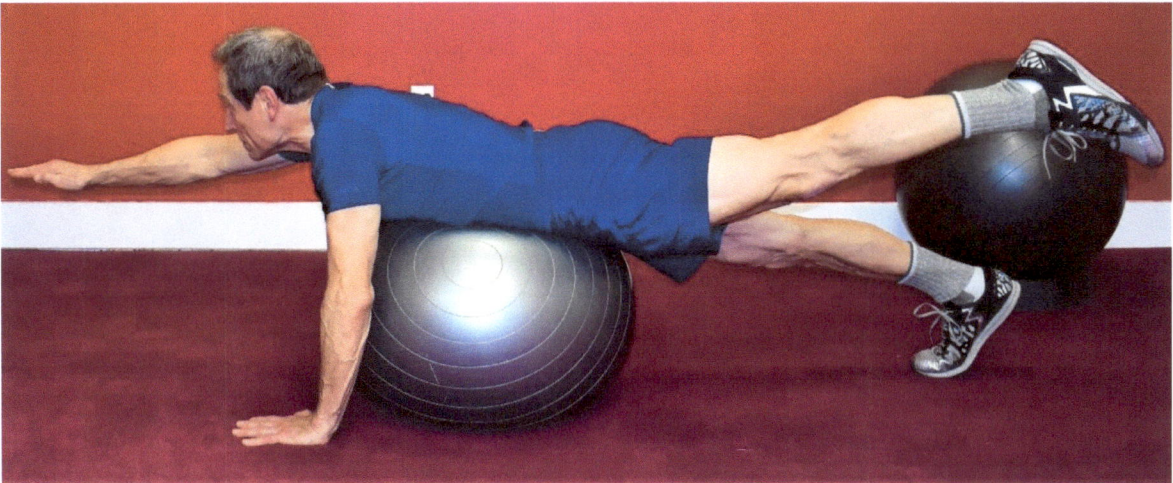

6. Great Blue Heron

a. Primary Target Muscles: Upper Erector Spinae/ Extensors of the Neck, Rhomboids, Trapezius, Posterior Deltoids, Long Head of the Triceps, Rotator Cuff Muscles, Lower Erector Spinae, Transverse Abdominis.

b. Performing abdominal exercises enables us to build strength in the flexor muscles of the torso. However, if we do not also develop flexible strength in the muscles that extend the thorax, shoulders, and neck, we will be saddled with increasingly stooped posture. Enter the Great Blue Heron, a simple but challenging exercise to reinforce postural elegance. As you execute each repetition of this exercise, imagine you are a heron flying through the mist rising from a lake early one morning. You feel the muscles between your shoulder blades pull your wings upward in preparation for their next downstroke.

c. Directions

(1) Lie face down with your lower sternum directly over the center of an agility ball. Your knees are straight. You feel a stretch in your hamstrings and calves. Your toes are dorsiflexed against the floor which creates a stretching sensation on the bottom of your feet and in your Achilles tendons. As you lower your head toward the floor, cross your arms in front of the ball, turn your hands and shoulders inward, and feel for a great stretch in the muscles between your scapulae and behind your shoulders. This is the Beginning Position (**Top**). Inhale and perform an abdominal vacuum.

(2) As you begin to exhale, raise your torso, head, and neck, lift your arms backward and upward, and rotate your shoulders and hands outward (**Middle**).

(3) As your upper torso rises from the ball, continue moving your shoulders backward and rotating them externally. When all target muscles feel tightly contracted, pause momentarily in the Peak Position (**Bottom**).

(4) Inhale and perform an abdominal vacuum as you lower your torso, head, shoulders, and arms to the beginning position.

(5) Repeat steps **(2)**-**(4)** for 10 invigorating repetitions.

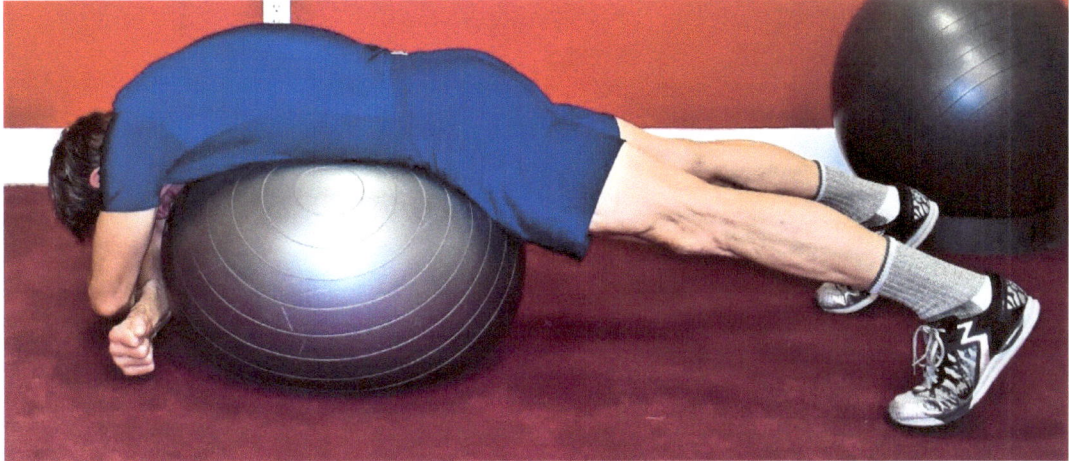

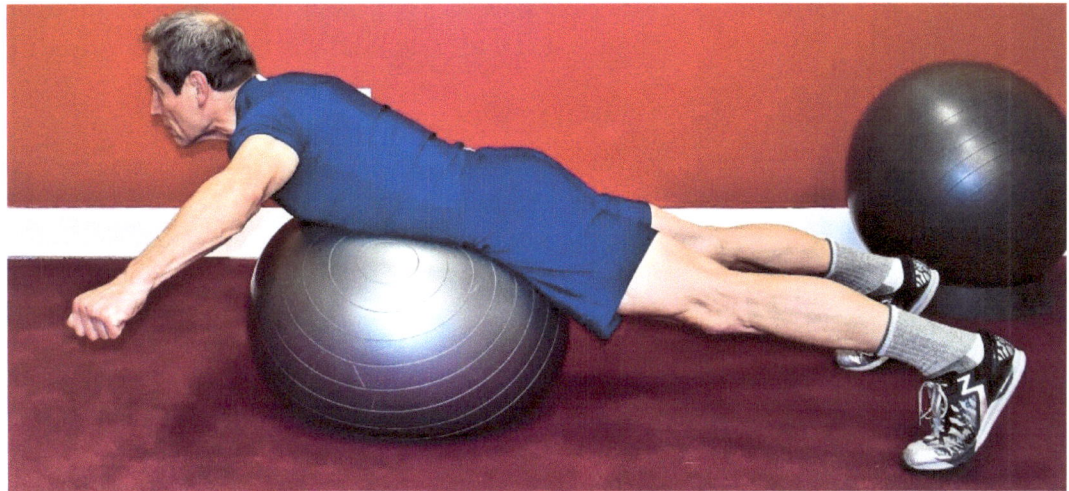

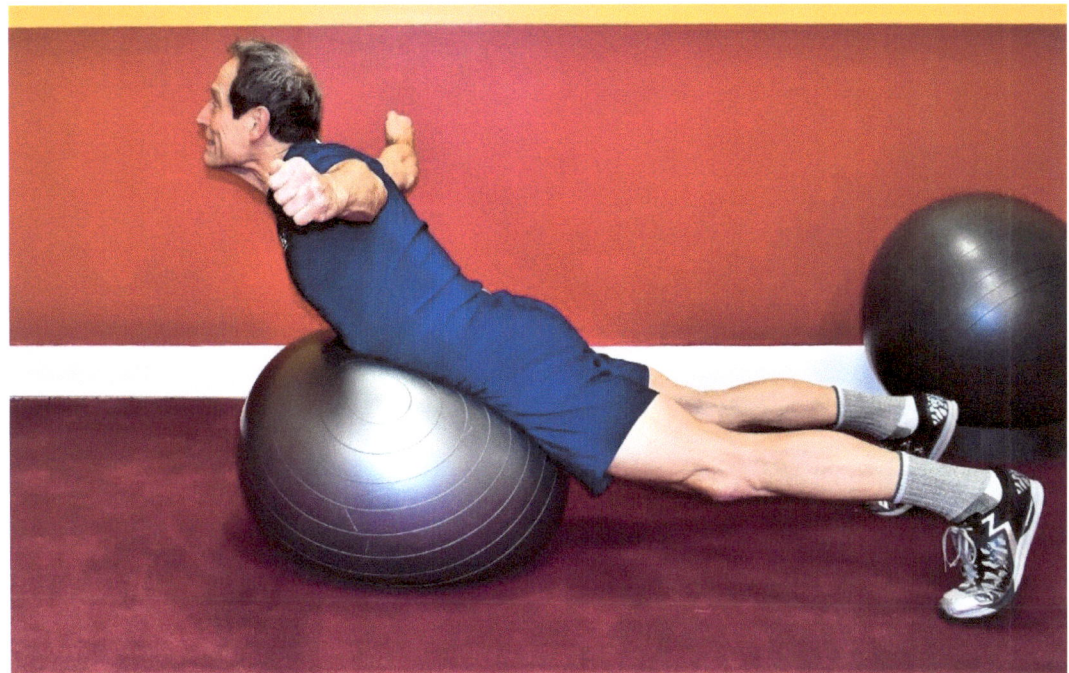

7. Inch Worm

   a. Target Muscle Groups: Hip Flexors and Rectus Abdominis

   b. This exercise is more important for developing whole-body agility and flexibility than it is for increasing the strength of specific muscle groups. In addition, it serves as excellent preparation for a more advanced exercise in an upcoming medley.

   c. c. Directions

(1) Kneel on the floor with an agility ball in front of your thighs. Lean forward, place your chest on the ball, and place your hands on the floor ahead. Next, roll forward and "walk" ahead on your hands until the ball is centered under the front of your thighs. Your hands are still on the floor in front of the ball, but your elbows are now fully extended. Extend your head and neck so you can see straight ahead and allow your chest to descend toward the floor. After performing an abdominal vacuum, you are in the Beginning Position (**Top**). Note how completely the abdomen is drawn up and in by the vacuum. Inhale.

(2) As you begin to exhale, use your lower rectus abdominis and hip flexors to bring your knees and the ball forward, as your torso rises, and your back rounds upward. As your knees bend, the ball will roll forward and contact your shins.

(3) Continue flexing your rectus abdominis muscles to pull your torso upward and your hips forward until you are kneeling atop the ball in the Peak Position (**Bottom**). Pause momentarily to savor the stretch in the muscles of your lower back.

(4) As you begin to inhale, perform an abdominal vacuum and allow your body to roll back to the beginning position. Pause momentarily.

(5) Repeat steps **(2)** to **(4)** for a total of 10 to 15 repetitions.

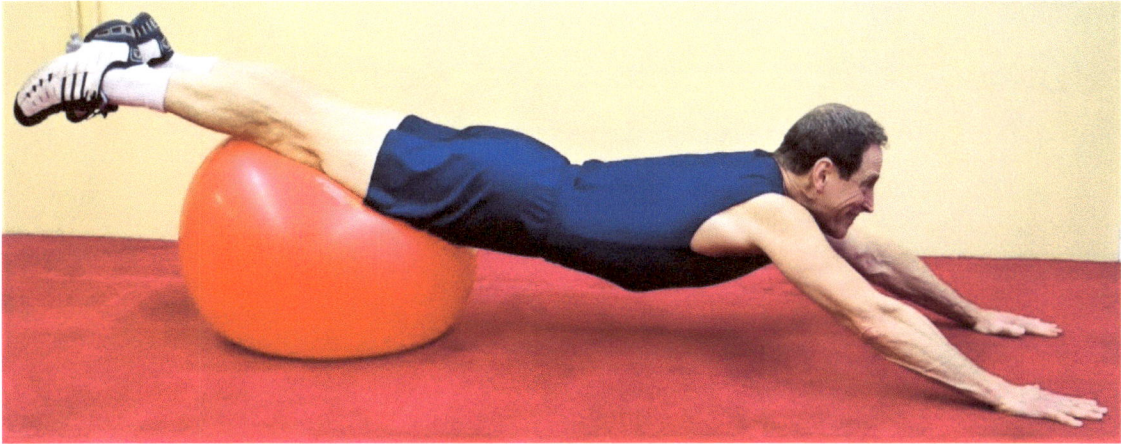

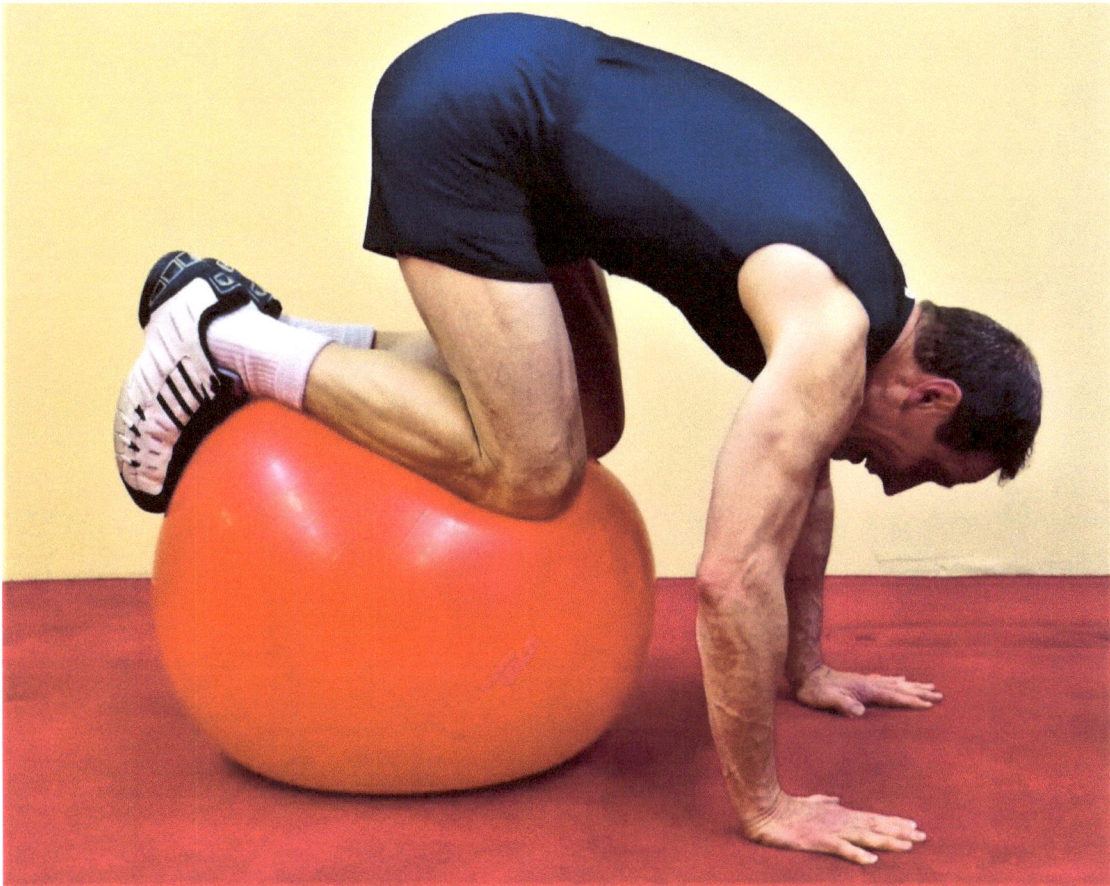

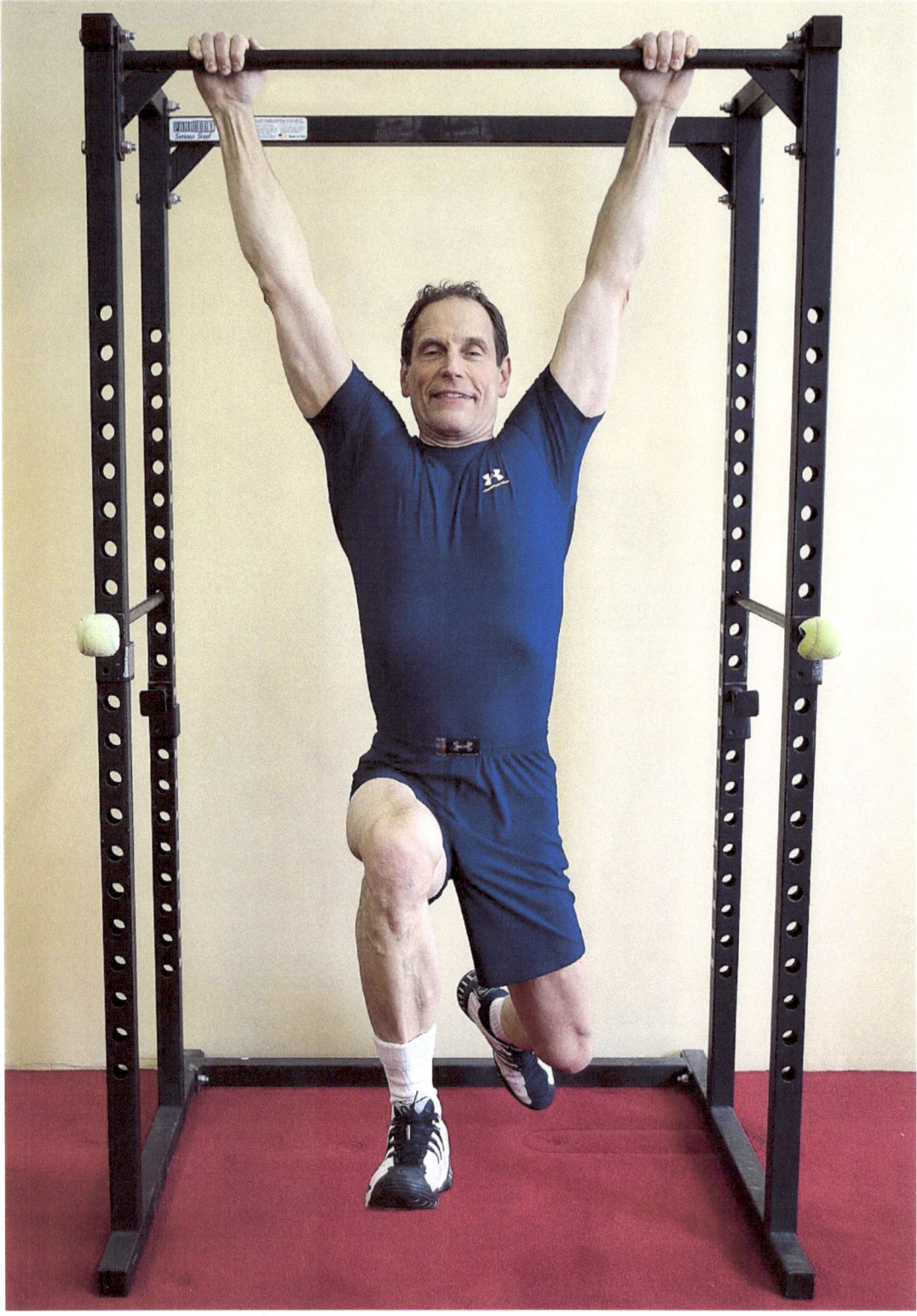

Chapter Three

Advanced Abdominal Medley #2

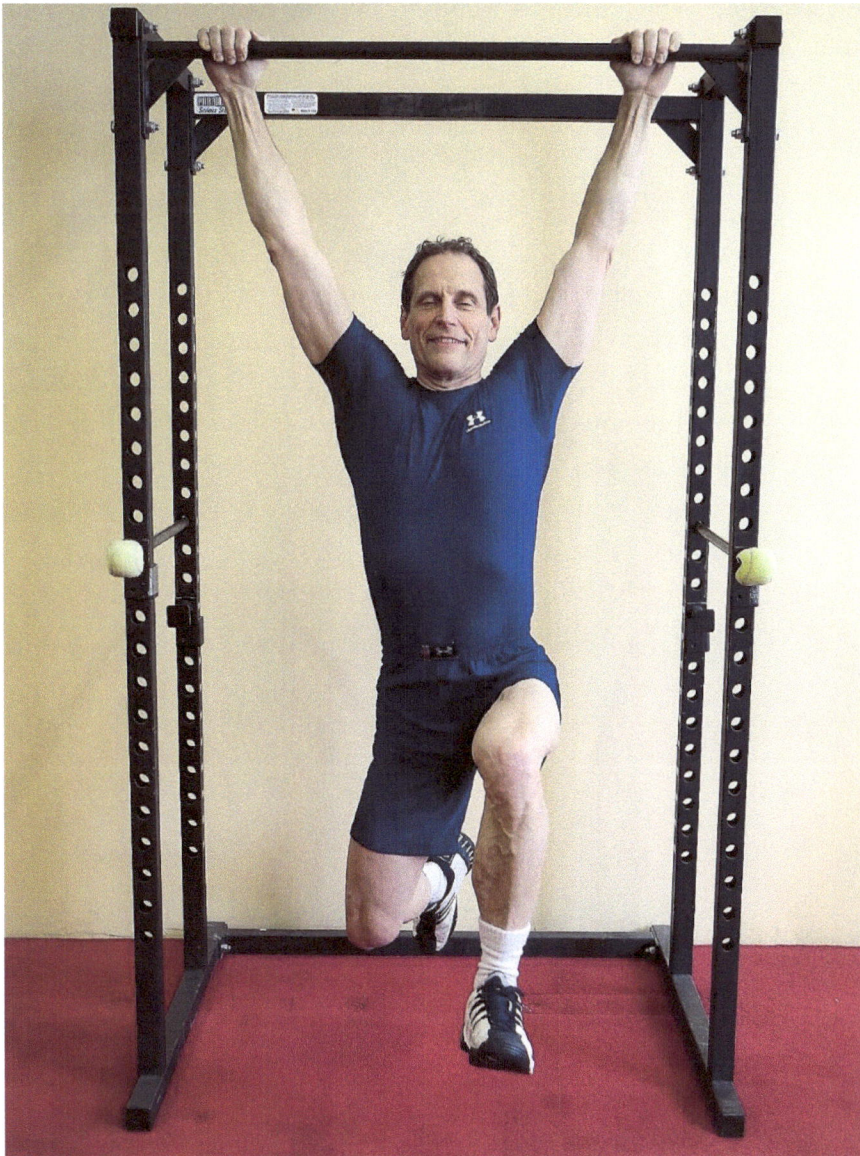

Advanced Abdominal Medley #2

1. Agility Ball Abdominal Curl/ Full Spine Extension w/ Weighted Ball

    a. Target Muscles: Lower & Upper Rectus Abdominis; Transverse Abdominis

    b. This exercise is a step above the Upper Abdominal Curl. We increase the range of motion in the target muscles by our placing hands overhead and adding a weighted medicine ball. Note: as you reach Peak Position, you have only raised your upper torso to be in line with the lower torso. This appears to make the exercise easier than curling your torso higher and further forward. However, flexing the torso too high allows the target muscles of the exercise to "take a break." When you raise your torso only to the point where it is even with your lower body, you feel much more intensive and continuous muscle tension in your rectus abdominis than you would by curling your torso higher and giving your target muscles an opportunity to relax momentarily in the middle of each repetition.

    c. Directions

        1) Holding a 5 to 10-pound medicine ball in your hands, put your arms over your head and recline backward over an agility ball. Your elbows are slightly bent. Continue to recline backward until you feel a moderate stretch over the entire length of your torso. This is the Beginning Position (**Top**). Do an abdominal vacuum, inhale, and pause.

        2) As you begin to exhale, initiate upward movement first by performing a lower abdominal curl into the ball. Continue curling your face and chest upward, but allow your arms and the ball to drag behind your head and chest. (**Middle**)

        3) Continue to curl your head, chest and arms upward until they reach a point where they are in line with your lower body. This is the Peak Position (**Bottom**). Pause briefly.

        4) Inhale, perform an abdominal vacuum, and return slowly to the beginning position. Enjoy 10-15 exhilarating repetitions.

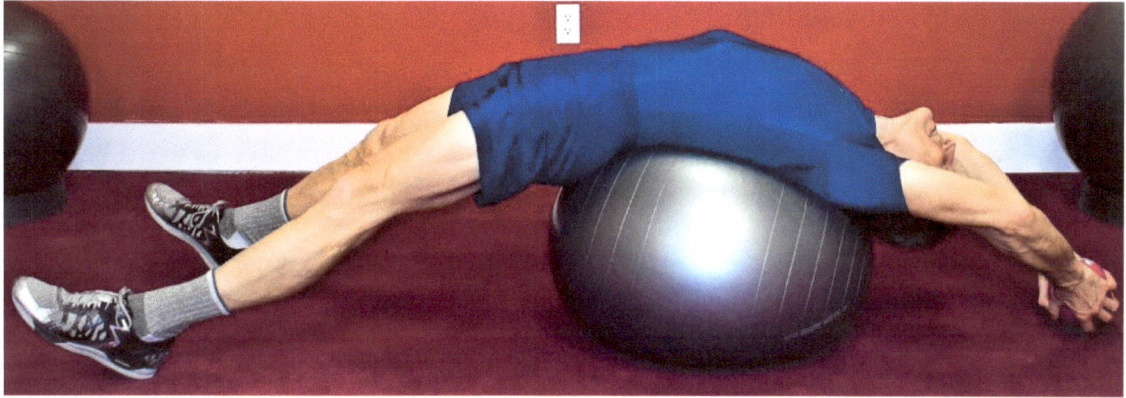

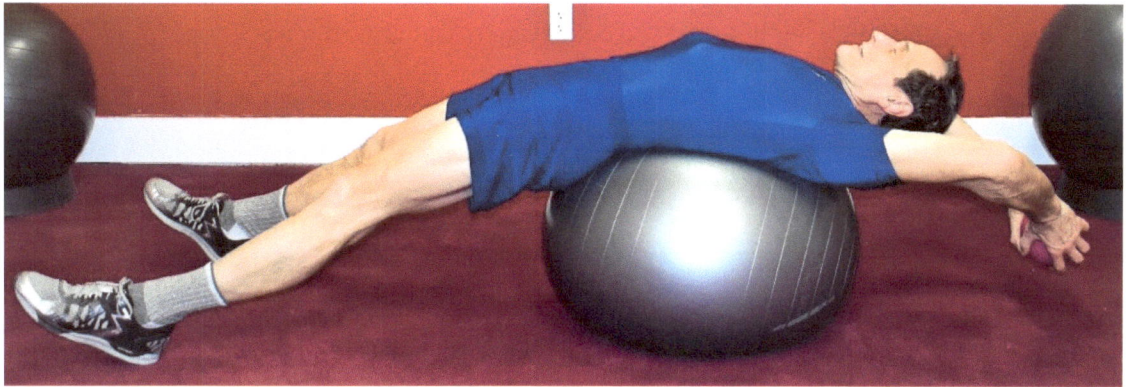

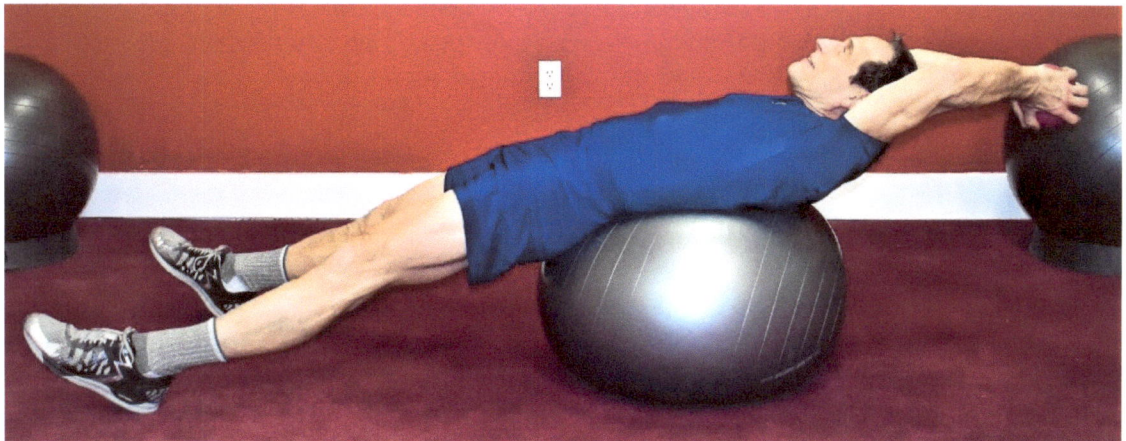

2. Reversely Rotating Side Jackknife w/ External Hip & Shoulder Rotation

   a. Target Muscles: Externally rotating muscles of the spine, hips, and shoulders; External and Internal Obliques; Neck and Rotator Cuff muscles.

   b. The wide ranges of simultaneous movements in this exercise enable us to develop the flexible strength and coordination we need to succeed in many different sports: tennis, baseball, archery, throwing the javelin etc.

   c. Directions

   1) With a 5# medicine ball in your right hand, lie on your left side with your left hip centered over an agility ball. Move your left foot forward from the ball approximately 12 inches, contacting the floor with the outside of your left shoe. Move your right foot backward approximately 12 inches and turn your hip and ankle inward, so the toes of your right shoe contact the floor.

   2) Allow your head, right upper torso, shoulder, and arm to move forward, down toward the floor, and then across your body until the until you feel a great stretch in all your target muscles. This is the Beginning Position (**Top**). You are looking directly at the floor.

   3) As with every advanced core exercise, do an abdominal vacuum before you initiate movement and then inhale.

   4) As you begin to exhale, pull the weighted ball and your outstretched right arm, backward, outward, and then upward toward the ceiling. Your head and neck turn rightward to a neutral position. At the same time, bring your right foot forward and upward while turning it outward (external rotation of the hip) as it rises toward the ceiling (**Middle**).

   5) Continue to exhale as you allow the weighted ball and your arm to move backward until you reach a position of a moderate stretch across your right shoulder and upper thorax. Meanwhile your right leg and foot have risen and turned outward. You are now facing the ceiling in the Peak Position (**Bottom**). Pause briefly and then inhale as you perform an abdominal vacuum and return to the beginning position.

   6) Perform 10-15 repetitions on this side and then enjoy an equal number while lying on your right side.

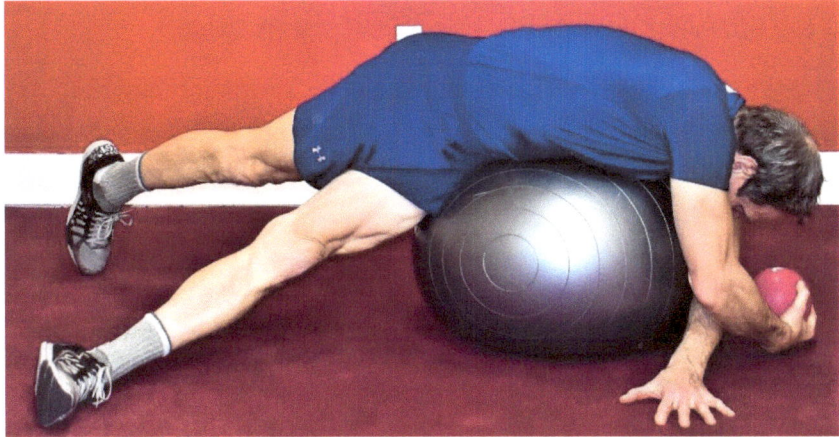

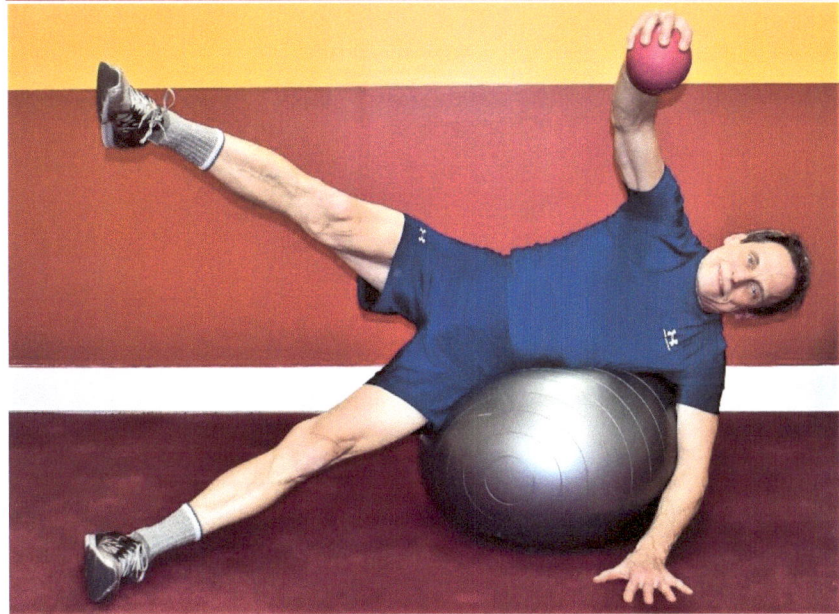

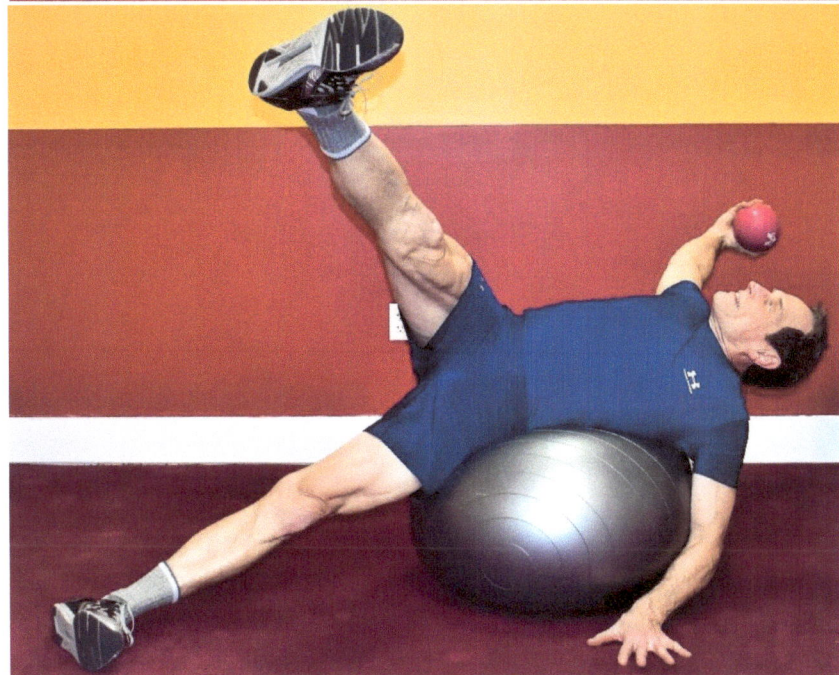

3. Forwardly Rotating Side Jackknife while Throwing Weighted Ball

a. Target Muscle Groups: Internal and External Rotators of the thorax, hips, shoulders, and neck. As advanced core exercises become more complex, it is increasingly difficult to name each specific target muscle group.

b. This exercise is almost a continuation of the previous one. Using a weighted ball is not only beneficial for those of us who want to throw with more power in our favorite sports. It also builds flexible shoulder strength for everyone who must put a suitcase in an over-the-seat storage bin or take down a heavy package from a high shelf. The ball pictured in this and the preceding exercise is a "slam ball", i.e. made to throw against a wall or floor without causing structural damage. It deforms when it strikes a hard surface, as you can see by viewing the elongated ball in the bottom photo.

c. Directions

1) Lie on your left side with the middle of your thorax over an agility ball. Your right leg is crossed over the left so the instep of your right shoe is 12 inches forward of the left. Your left arm is extended forward with your left hand on the floor. Meanwhile, your right arm and shoulder are extended straight backward, until you feel a stretch across your chest, which is enhanced by the weight of a 5# slam ball in your right hand. Your head and neck are turned toward the ceiling. This is the Beginning Position (**Top**). Do an abdominal vacuum and inhale.

2) As you begin to exhale, externally rotate and abduct your right hip and simultaneously raise the slam ball forward and upward, using a throwing type of motion with your right arm and shoulder. Meanwhile, your neck is rotating to the left. This is the midline position (**Middle**).

3) Continue to exhale as you bring the slam ball further forward and then downward toward the floor, releasing your grip on the ball as you do. Simultaneously, your right leg and hip rotate inward, backward, and downward until the toes of your right shoe impact the floor at the same time as the ball and your head turns fully to left so that you are looking directly at the floor (**Bottom**). Note the prominent neck muscle contractions, demonstrating why strong neck muscles are essential for successful performance of advanced core exercises.

4) Grab the ball, inhale, and perform an abdominal vacuum as you return to the beginning position. Enjoy 10 dynamic repetitions on each side.

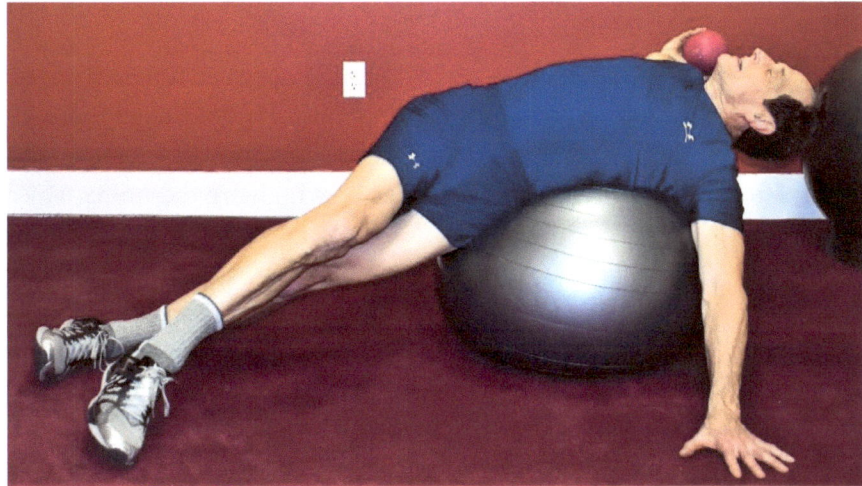

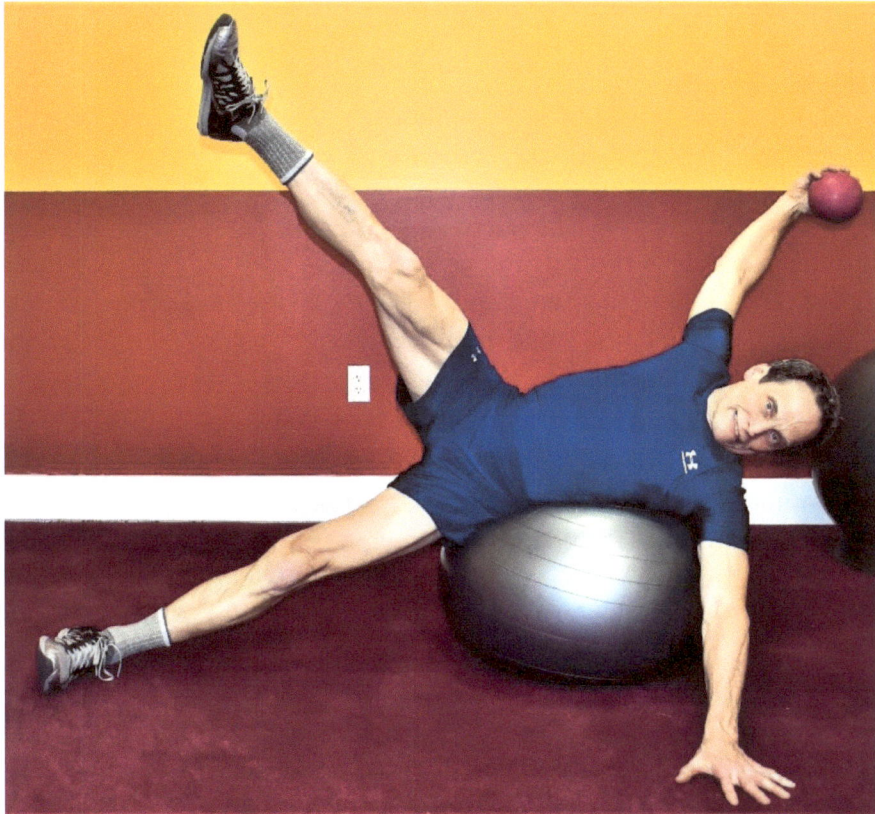

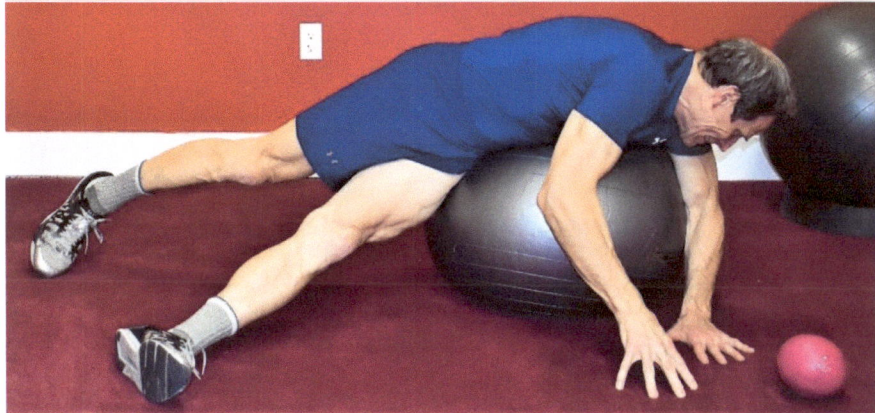

4. Drawbridge

a. Target Muscles: Lower and Upper Rectus Abdominis; Hip and Shoulder Extensors and Flexors.

b. This exercise is a major step forward in difficulty and excitement from the Inch Worm in the previous medley. Perfecting this exercise helps us to develop ever-greater whole-body flexibility, balance, coordination, and agility, elements of health which are the objectives of Strength for Life® training.

c. Directions

1) Kneeling upon the floor with an agility ball immediately in front of your knees, lean your chest and torso onto the ball and roll forward. Continue to move your body forward until your knees are as straight as possible and directly above the center of the ball. Simultaneously, stretch your arms, shoulders, and hands forward until your elbows are fully straightened as you touch the floor. Keep your head up and your eyes looking ahead. This is the Beginning Position (**Top**). If your lower spinal complex is strong and healthy, you should feel a pleasing sense of extension, but no pain, in your lower back. Perform an abdominal vacuum and inhale.

2) As you begin to exhale, use your rectus abdominis and hip flexors to pull your legs forward and your torso upward slowly. Keep your knees straight as they lose contact with the ball.

3) Continue exhaling as you move your whole body forward and your gluteals upward until you feel the weight of your upper body is almost directly above your hands and shoulders. Your knees are still straight, so you feel a great stretch in your hamstrings, while your abdominal muscles feel tightly contracted. This is the Peak Position (**Bottom**). You have raised the deck of the bridge so high that even the Tall Ships can pass safely below.

4) Pause momentarily in the Peak Position, then initiate an abdominal vacuum as you inhale and descend slowly to the beginning position. Enjoy no more than 10 repetitions of this exhilarating exercise. More is not better. Better is better.

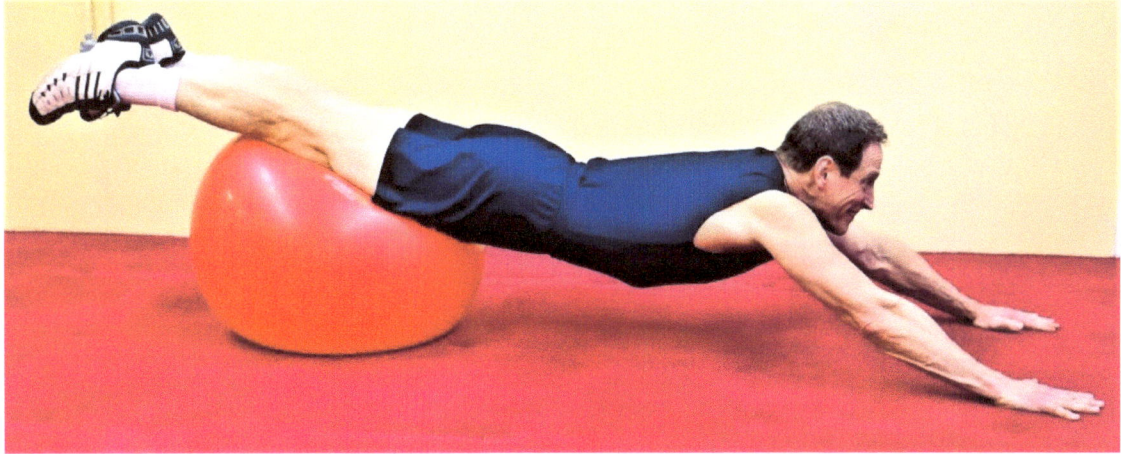

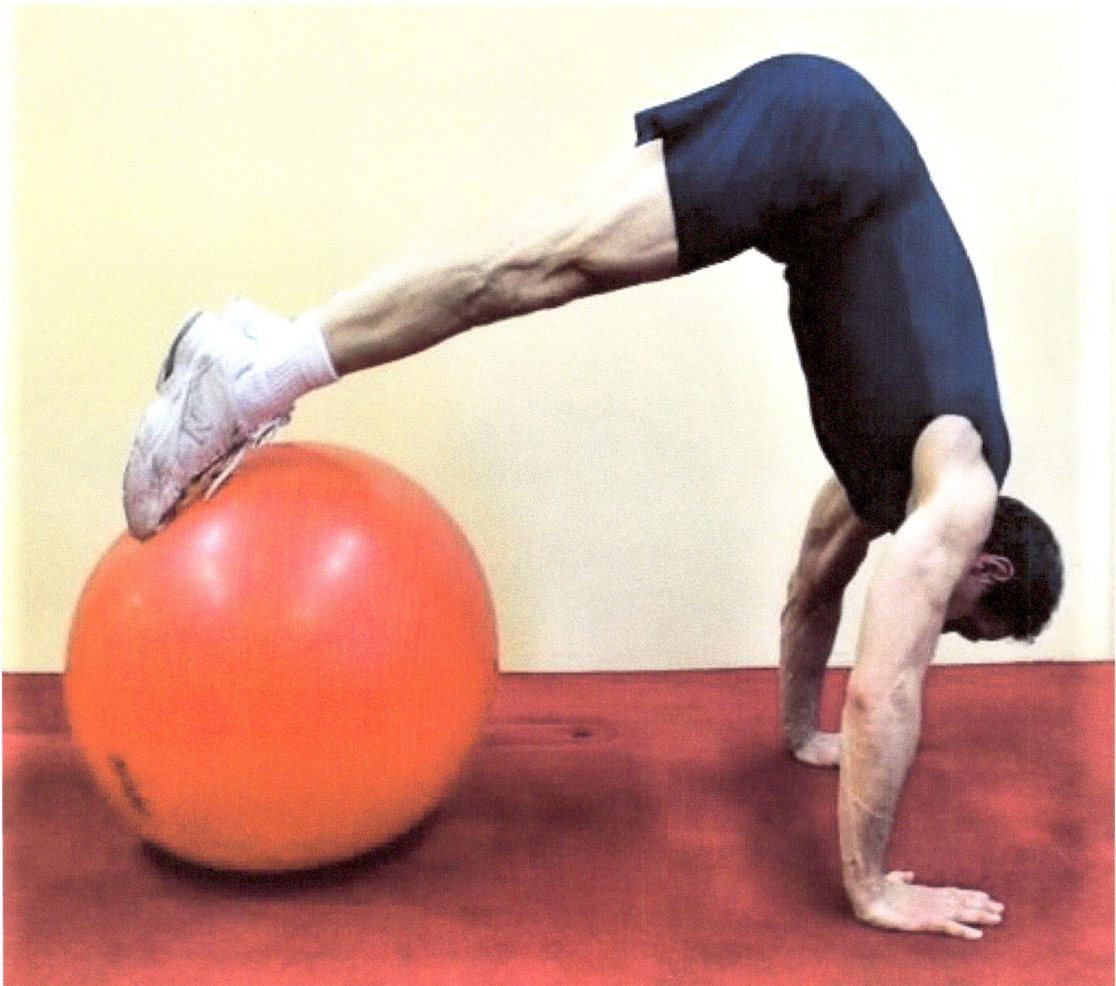

5. Gluteus Maximus Curl

a. Target Muscles: Gluteus Maximus, Erector Spinae, Iliopsoas.

b. This is the equivalent of performing Backups (exercise #6 in Medley #3 of *AbSfl!* Volume 1) one leg at a time, creating stronger contractions in the gluteus maximus than in the erector spinae. This exercise is also great for increasing the range of motion of the sacroiliac joints and stretching the Iliopsoas muscles.

c. Directions

(1) Lie face down with your chest and abdomen across a flat bench. Grasp the side of the bench to hold your torso firmly in place. With your knees bent at 90 degrees, allow your hips and lower extremities to hang down the opposite side of the bench. This is the Beginning Position (**Top**). Perform and Abdominal Vacuum and inhale.

(2) Exhale as you raise your left thigh upward until you feel a strong contraction in your left gluteus maximus (**Middle).** Pause briefly.

(3) Inhale as you slowly lower your left thigh to the beginning position. Pause.

(4) Exhale as you raise you right thigh by contracting your right gluteus maximus maximally. Pause in this Peak Position (**Bottom).**

(5) Inhale as you return to the beginning position. Continue alternately contracting your left and right glutes until you have enjoyed 10 repetitions on each side.

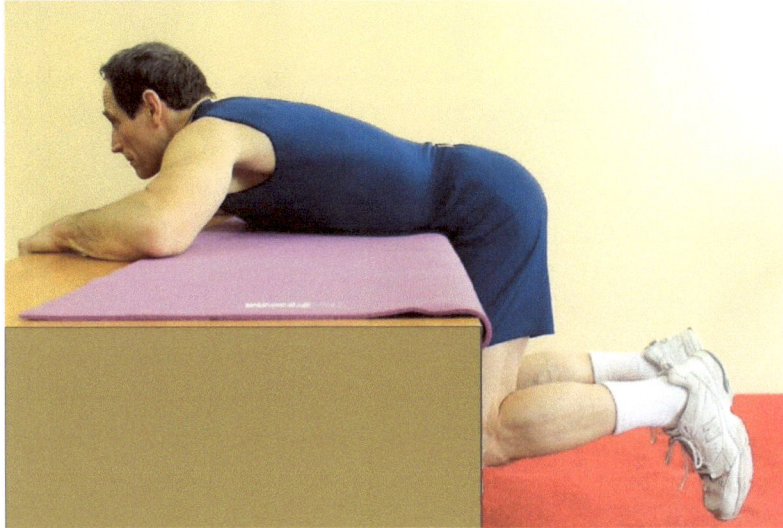

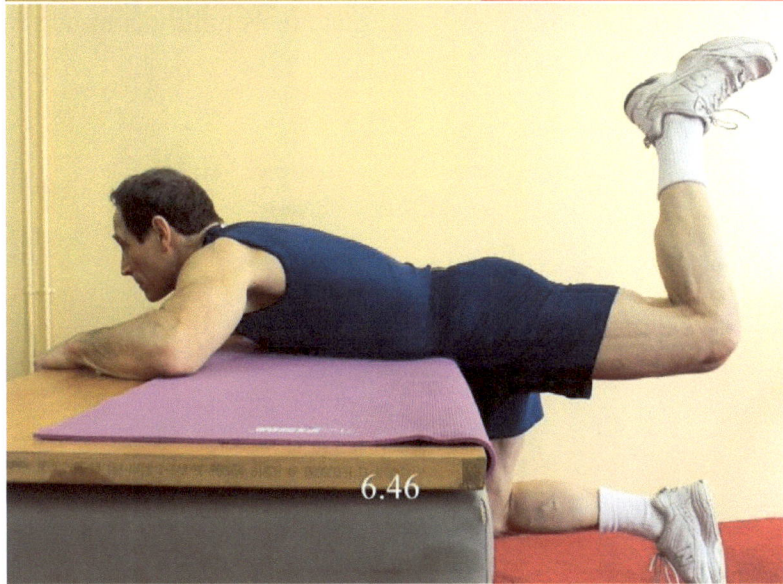

6.46

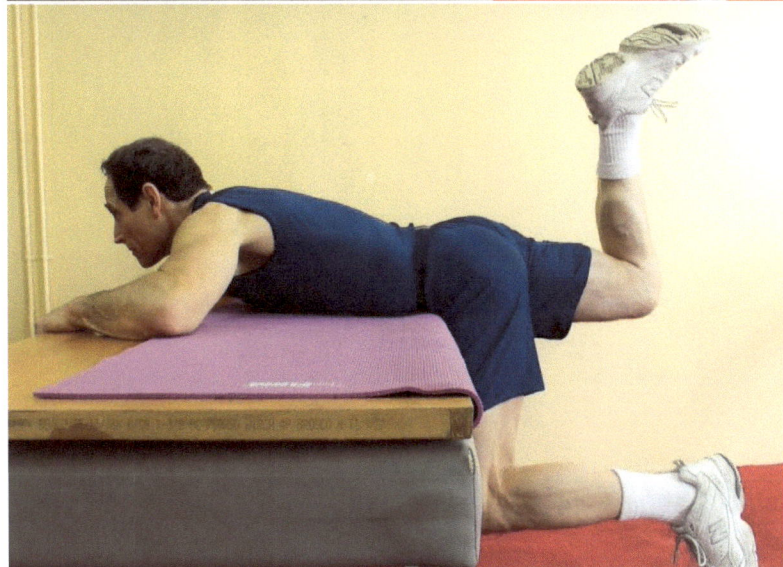

6. Running in Air

   a. Target Muscle Groups: Flexors and Extensors of the hip

   b. A great exercise to develop flexible strength in the hip muscles, increase   sacroiliac and shoulder flexibility, and to lengthen of your running stride.

   c. **c**. Directions

(1) Hang from a chinning bar with an overhand grip and your elbows straight. Bend both knees to 90° and point them toward the floor. After you perform an abdominal vacuum, you are in the Beginning Position (**This page below**). Inhale.

(2) As you begin to exhale, flex your left knee upward and forward until your left thigh is parallel with the floor. Simultaneously, extend your right hip backward until you feel a strong contraction in your right gluteus maximus and a great stretch in your right groin area (**Top next page**). Pause momentarily and inhale.

(3) Exhale as you reverse sides, flexing your right hip until your thigh reaches 90° in front you while extending your left hip behind until that glute feels tightly contracted (**Bottom**

(4) Continue to alternate flexing and extending your hips slowly until you have savored 10 repetitions on each side.

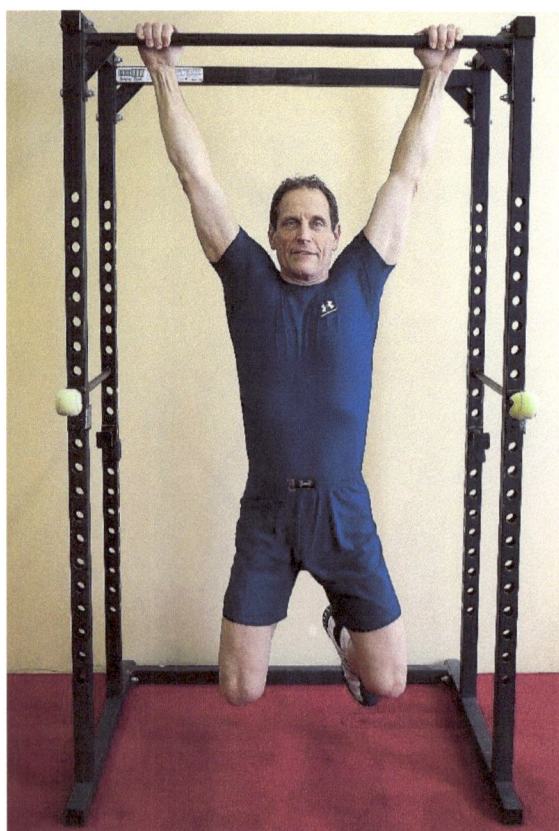

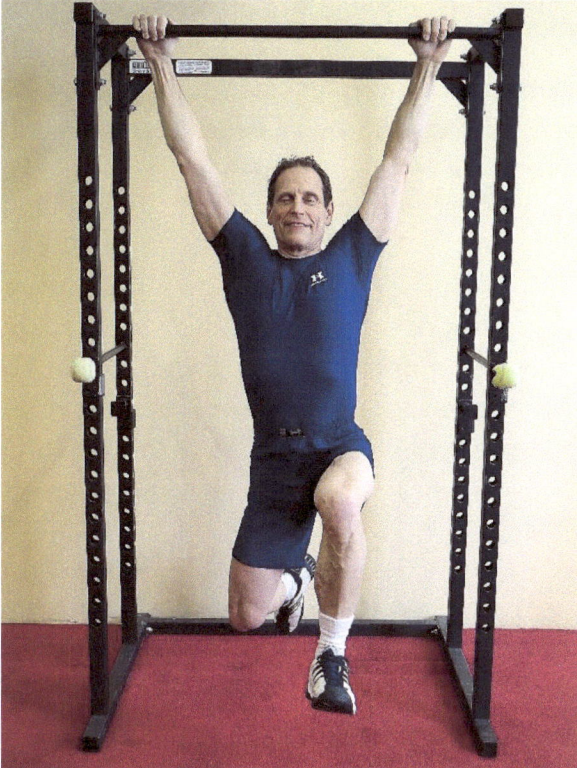

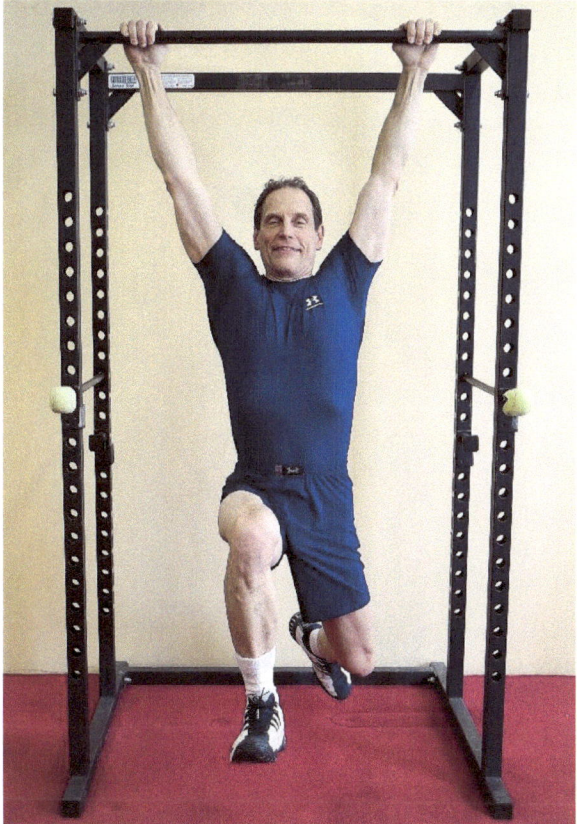

7. Paratrooper: Whole-Body Extensions on a Bench

   a. Target Muscles: Extensors of the Back, Neck, and Hips; External Rotators and Retractors of the Shoulders; Dorsiflexors and Plantar Flexors of the Ankle

   b. This exercise builds tremendous strength in the muscles of the spine and hips. Note that in the Beginning Position the ankles are dorsiflexed to stretch the Achilles tendons and that the shoulders are rotated internally.

   c. Directions

   1) Lie face down on a flat weight bench, allowing your head to stretch downward. With your knees straight, allow your legs to descend toward the floor behind you on each side of the bench. Cross your elbows in front of you and rotate your shoulders internally, so you feel a great stretch between your shoulder blades. With your knees still straight, raise your toes in the direction of your kneecaps, until you feel a terrific stretch in your Achilles tendons. You should feel a great stretch up and down your entire body. This is the Beginning Position (**Top**). As always, do an abdominal vacuum and inhale.

   2) As you begin to exhale, very slowly raise your entire body upward toward the ceiling and rotate your shoulders externally. You will feel a gradually increasing tension in all the muscle of your spine, shoulders, and hips (**Middle**).

   3) Continue to elevate your entire body as high as your brain tells you is safe, that is, until you feel the target muscles of your spine, shoulders, and hips are tightly contracted. In the Peak Position you should feel as though your whole body is ready to take flight (**Bottom**).

   4) Begin to inhale as you allow your body to descend slowly to the Beginning Position. As you do, perform another abdominal vacuum.

   5) Enjoy performing 10 repetitions.

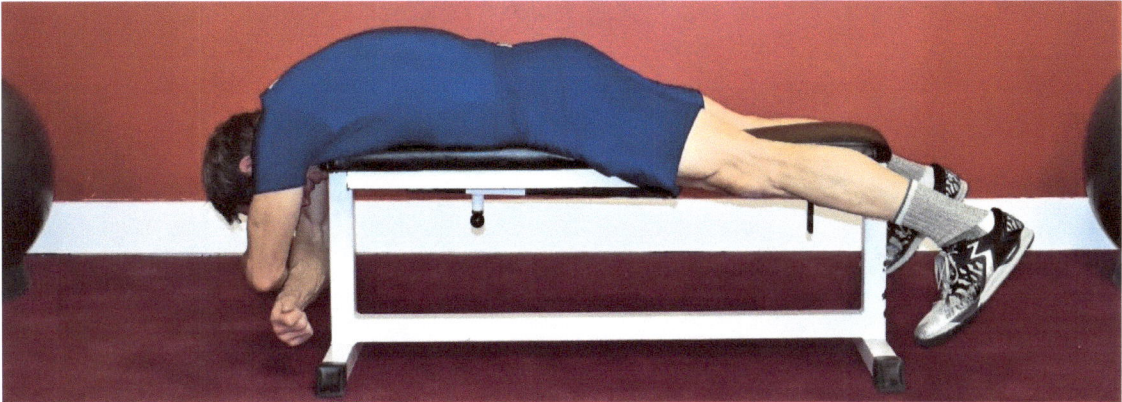

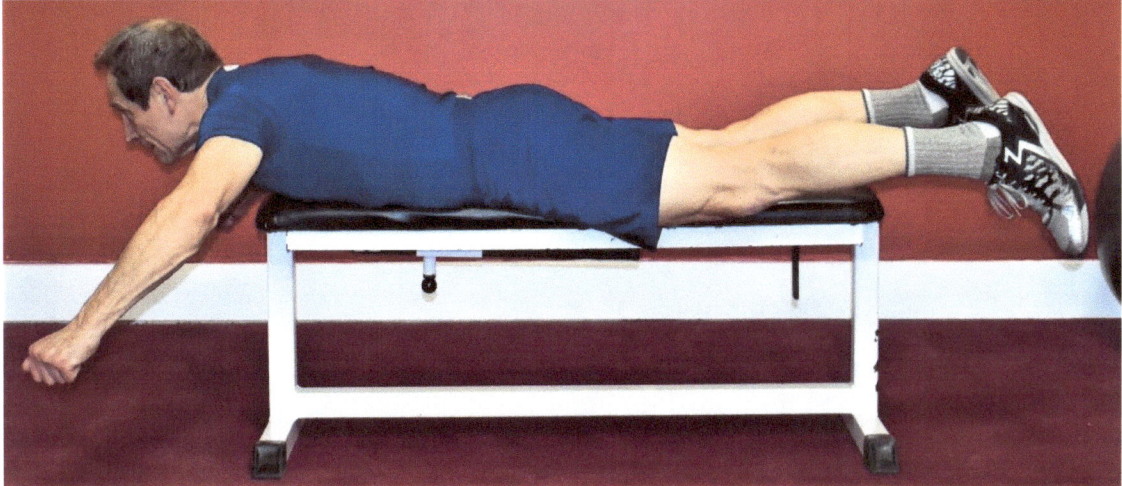

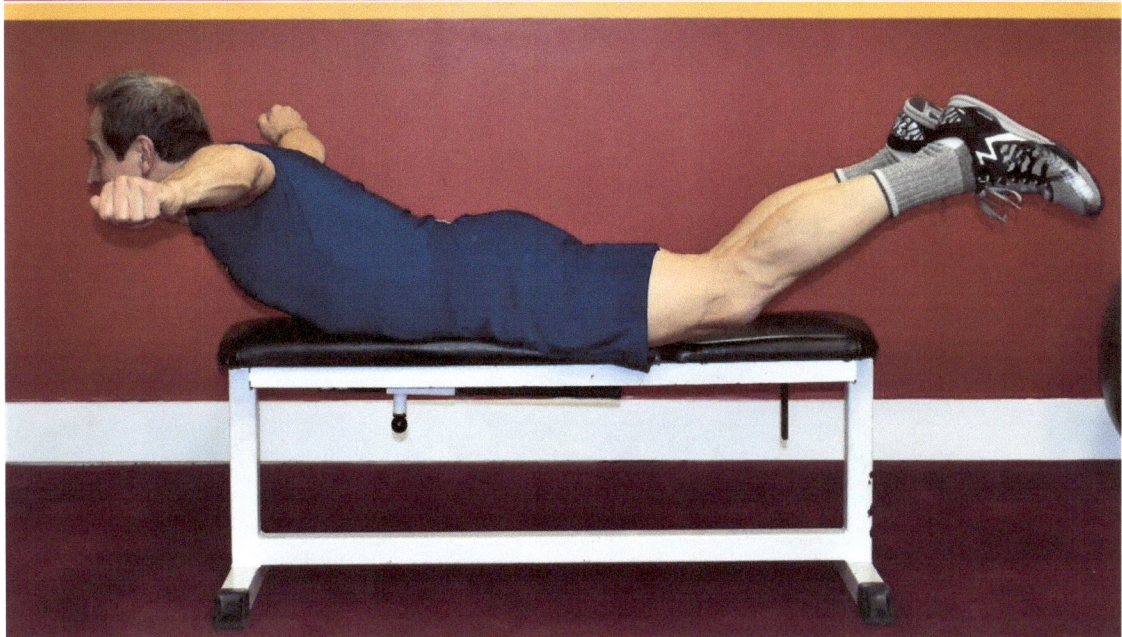

41

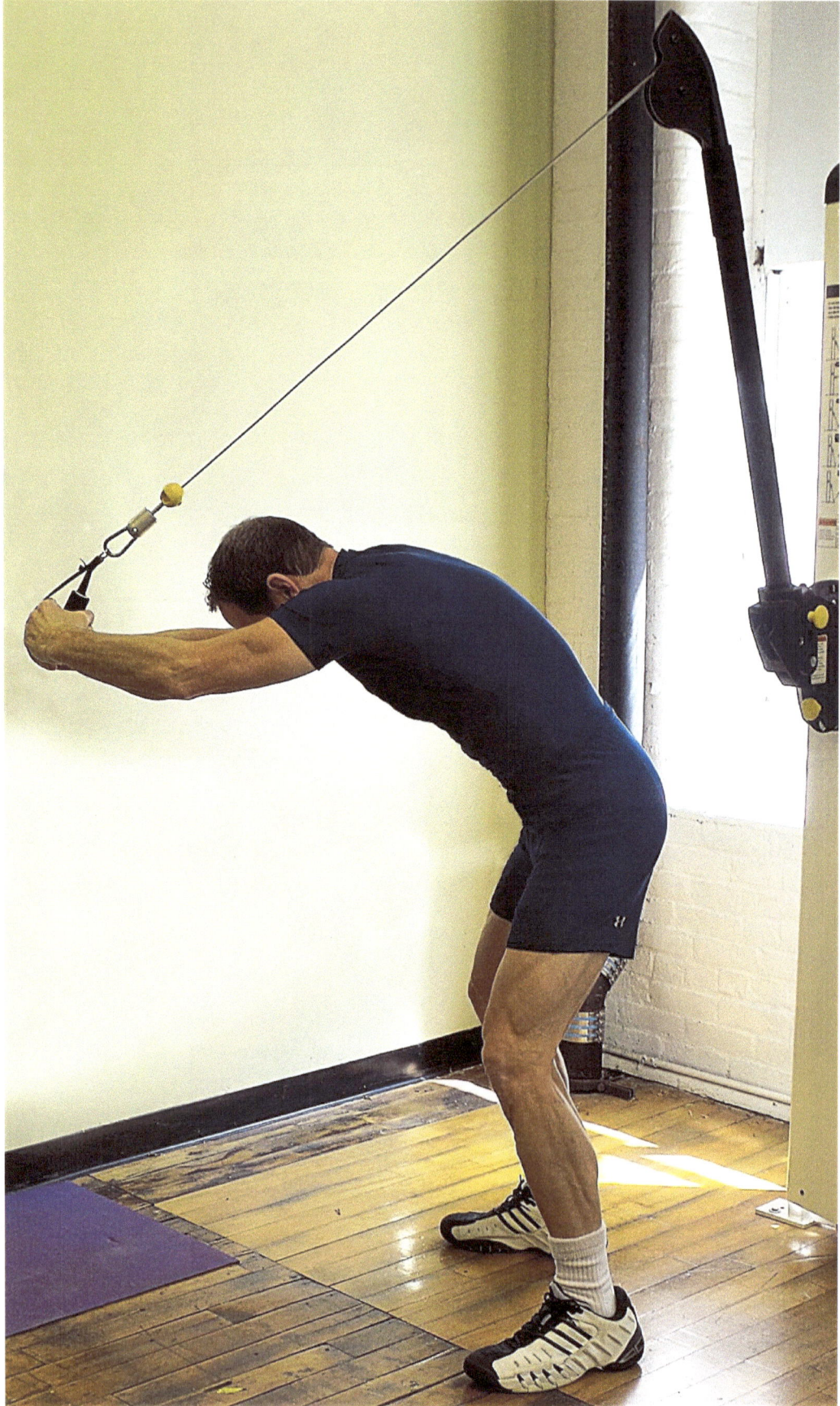

Chapter Four

Advanced Abdominal Medley # 3

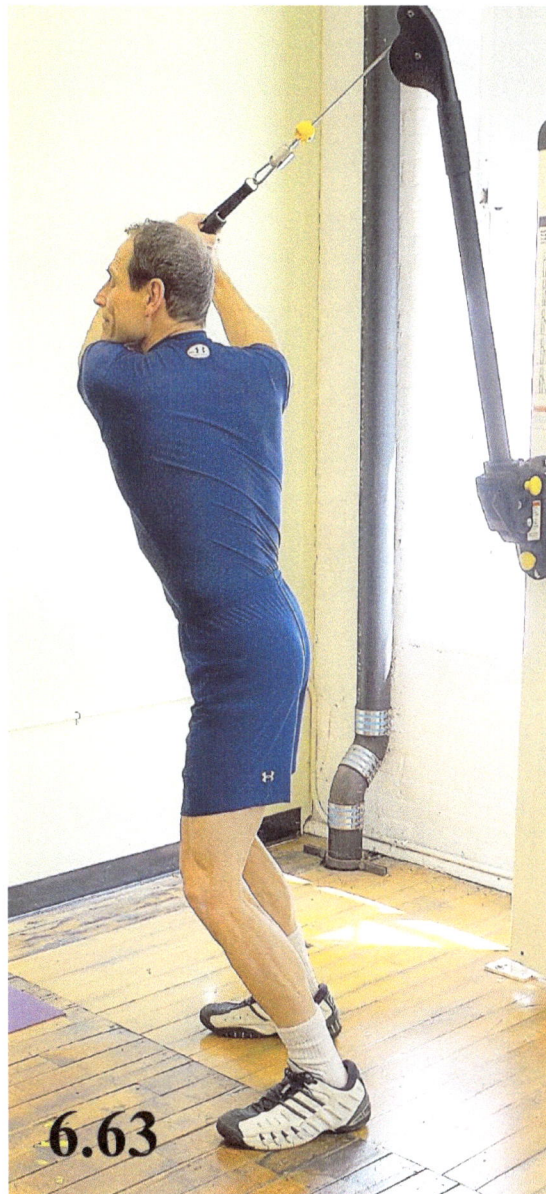

6.63

1. Ring the Bell at the Fair (Standing Abdominal Cable Curl)

   a. Primary Target Muscles: Rectus Abdominis; Transverse Abdominis

   b. In a state fair tradition, we simulate swinging a mallet from overhead, hitting an impact plate, and propelling a metal disc upward to clang the bell at the top of a pole. In this exercise, curl your torso downward only about 45^0-60^0, leaving the impact and the ringing bell to our imaginations.

   c. c. Directions

   (1) Using a moderate weight, stand with your back to an overhead cable, grasp the handle overhead, and walk forward until your lats and abdominals feel stretched. With your knees and elbows bent slightly, you are in the Beginning Position (**This page below**). Inhale.

   (2) As you begin to exhale, do abdominal vacuum, a lower abdominal curl, then an upper abdominal curl. Use your abdominals, not your arms and shoulders, to bring the mallet down (**Top next page**).

   (3) Continue curling down and forward until your abdominals feel tightly contracted in the Peak Position (**Bottom**). Pause.

   (4) Perform an abdominal vacuum and inhale slowly as you uncurl to the beginning position. Enjoy 10 superb repetitions.

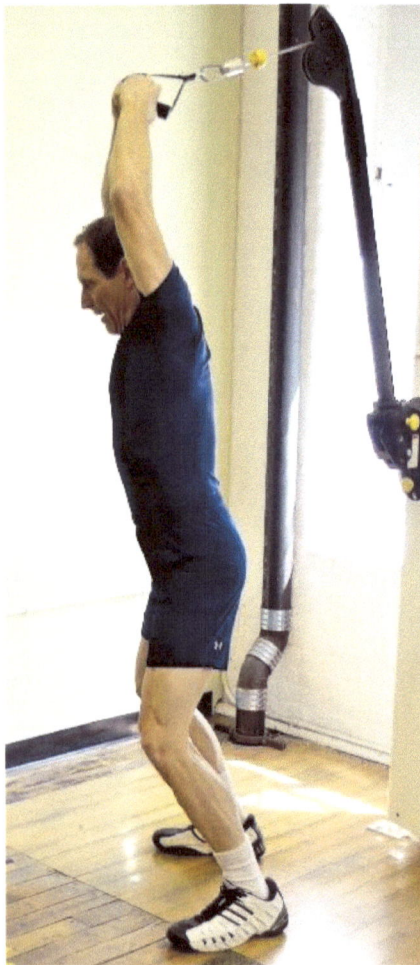

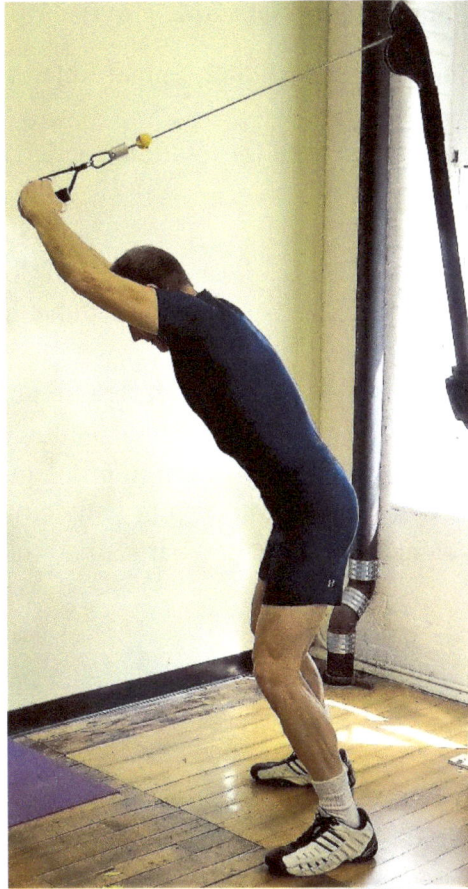
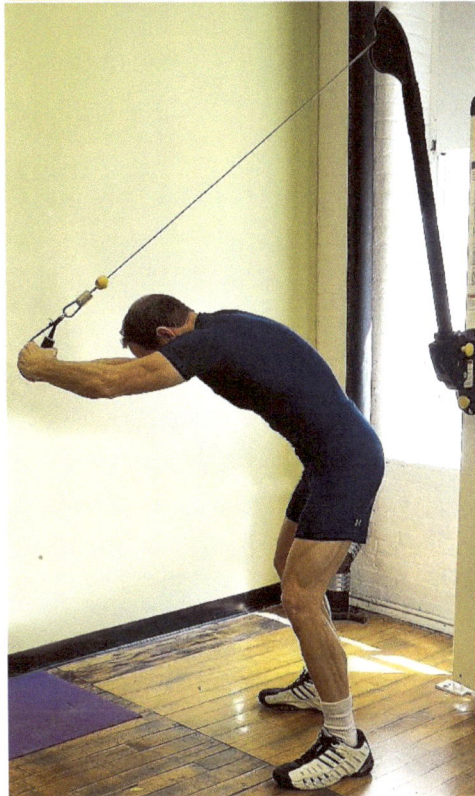

2. Woodchopper (Standing Diagonal Abdominal Cable Curl)

a. Target Muscles: External and Internal Obliques, Spinal Rotators, Rectus Abdominis, Transverse Abdominis, Serratus Anterior, Lat. Dorsi

b. This exercise creates the strength we need for rotational actions, such as raking, tennis, or golf. Use a moderate weight.

c. Directions

(**1**) Stand with your back to an overhead cable and move two feet to your left. Turn to the right, reach over your right shoulder, grasp the handle with both hands, do an abdominal vacuum, and inhale (**6.63**).

(**2**) Exhale as you turn your upper body slowly from right to left and downward. **6.64** is the halfway point. Continue rotating your torso and shoulders down and to the left until your hands reach the midline of your body in the Peak Position (**6.65**). Pause.

(**3**) Inhale and perform an abdominal vacuum as your body unwinds slowly to the Beginning Position. Do 10 repetitions right to left, change your stance, and then 10 superb repetitions left to right.

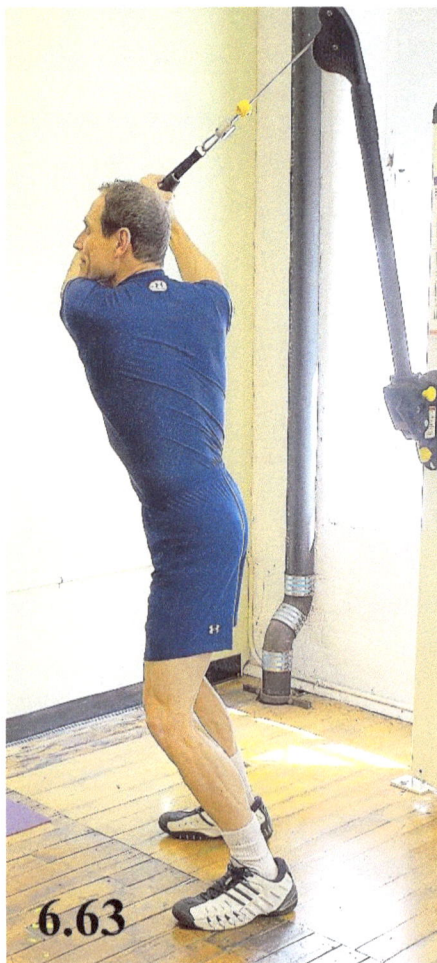

6.63

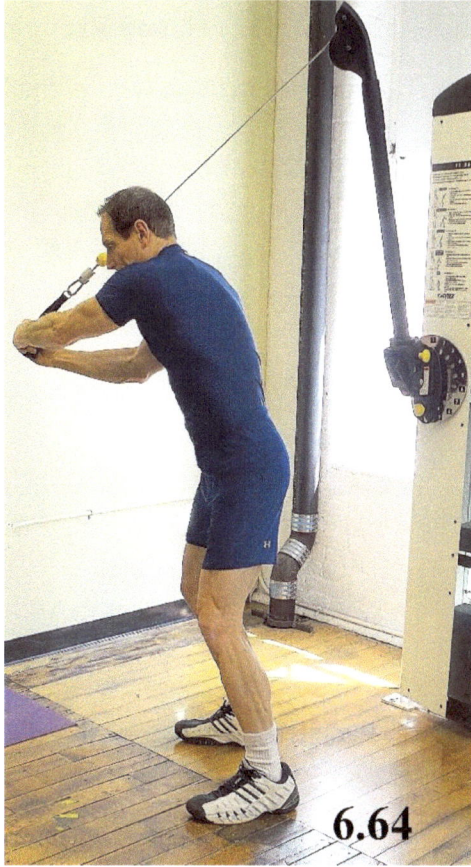

6.64

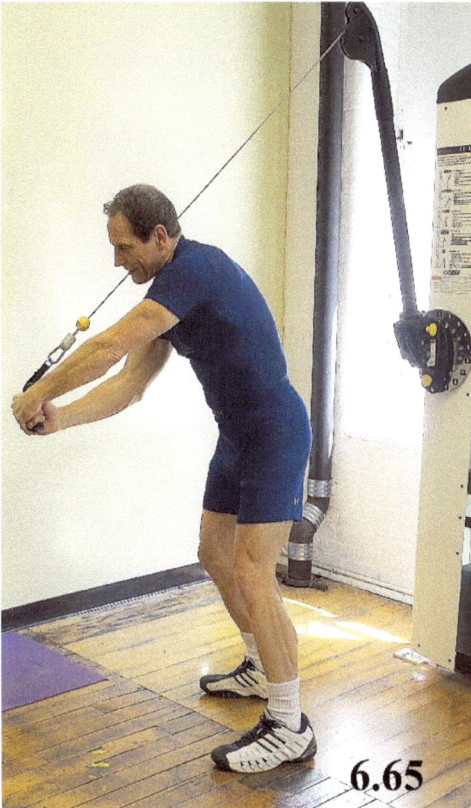

6.65

3. Hanging Double Bent Knee Raise, Abdominal Curl, and Vacuum

a. Target Muscles: Lower and Upper Rectus Abdominis, Hip and Neck Flexors and Extensors, Transverse Abdominis

b. This and the two following exercises are performed while gripping a chin-up bar. If your grip strength is insufficient to hold your body weight for 10 repetitions, do as many as you can, take a break, do a few more, etc., until you have completed ten. Very soon you will be able to sustain your body weight for ten exciting repetitions, which means your grip strength will have increased as well. In doing these hanging exercises, you will feel a great stretch in your shoulders.

c. Directions

(1) Grasp the bar with an overhand grip.

(2) Flex your knees to 90° so they point toward the floor while the soles of your shoes are aimed directly behind you. Allow the weight of your body to hang toward the floor, supported solely by the flexors of your hands and forearms. Enjoy the stretch in your shoulders.

(3) Tilt your head backward and look up and as far back as your brain tells you is safe for your neck. Do an abdominal vacuum as you inhale. This is the Beginning Position (**Top**).

(4) As you begin to exhale, initiate upward movement of your lower torso by performing a lower abdominal curl. Continue with an upper abdominal curl as you raise your knees slowly toward your chest while flexing your head forward and downward.

(5) When your thighs are approximately parallel to the floor and your abdominal and neck flexor muscles feel tightly contracted, pause momentarily in the Peak Position (**Bottom**).

(6) As you begin to inhale, slowly lower your knees, extend your head and neck backward, and do a slow abdominal vacuum until you reach the Beginning Position. Pause momentarily.

(7) Repeat Steps (4) to (6) for 10 exhilarating repetitions.

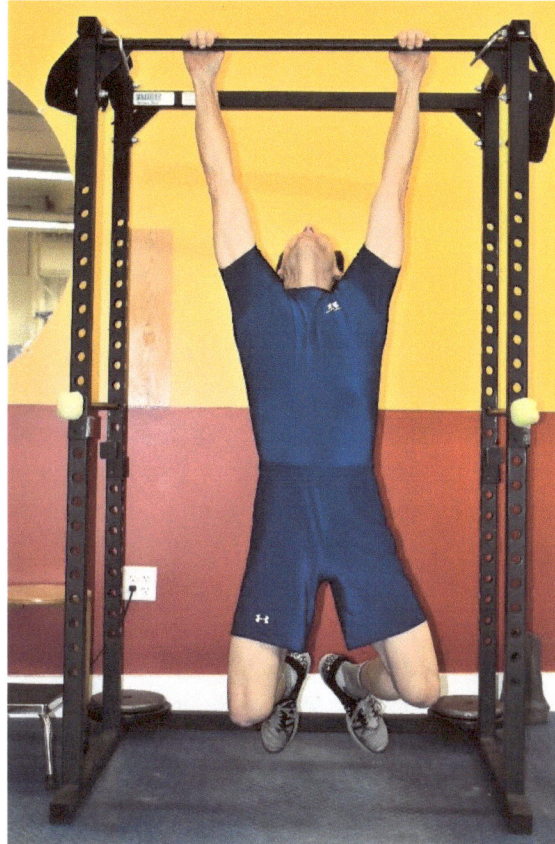

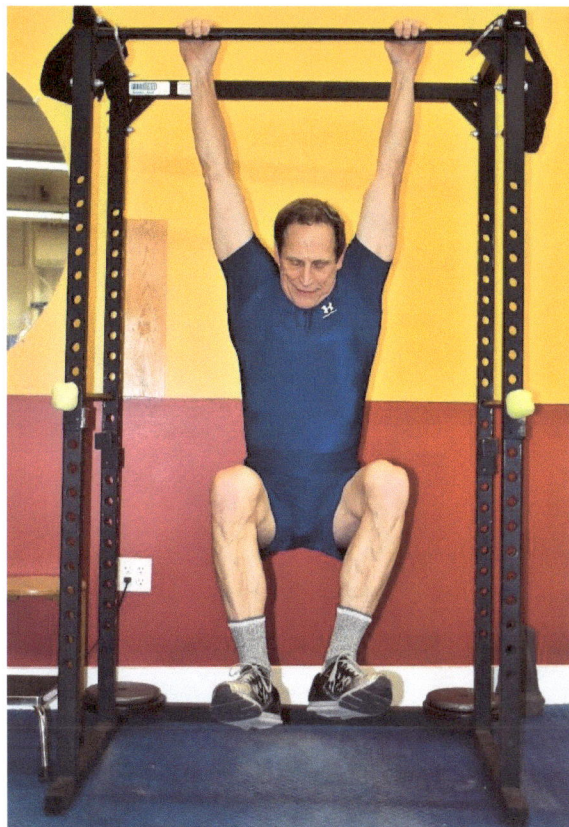

4. Hanging Hip Hiker

    a. Target Muscles: Quadratus Lumborum (AKA:" Hip Hiker Muscle"), Lateral Obliques, Hip Abductors

    b. We use these muscles to dance, walk, even to get in and out of a car.

    c. Directions

        1) Hang from a chinning bar with your knees bent at 90°. Looking straight ahead, perform an abdominal vacuum and inhale. This is the Beginning Position (**This page below**).

        2) As you begin to exhale, slowly raise your right hip sideways and upward to the right. Pause. Feel full contractions in the muscles on the right side of your lower torso/hip complex and a great stretch in the corresponding muscles on the left lower torso. Pause completely in the Peak Position (**Top next page**).

        3) As you inhale, do an abdominal vacuum, and return to the Beginning Position. Pause again.

        4) Exhale and perform the same movements of steps **(2)-(3)** to the left (**Bottom next page**). Perform 10 repetitions to each side.

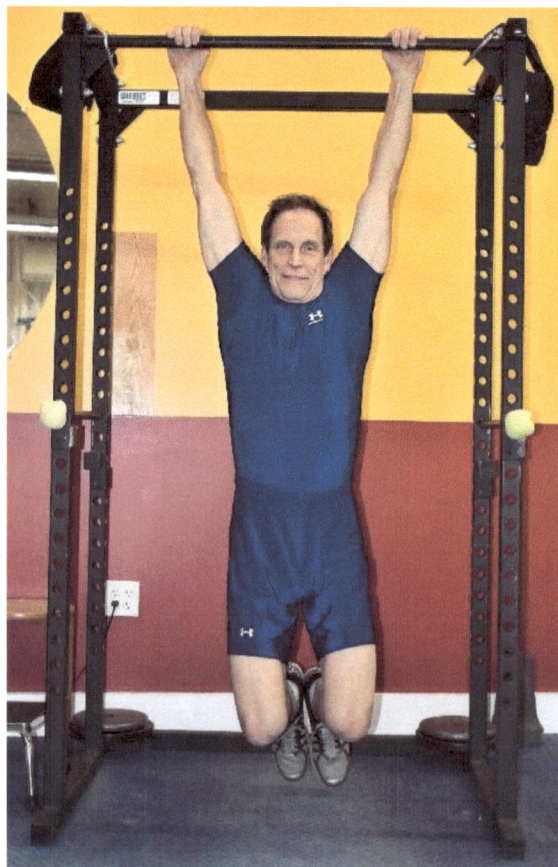

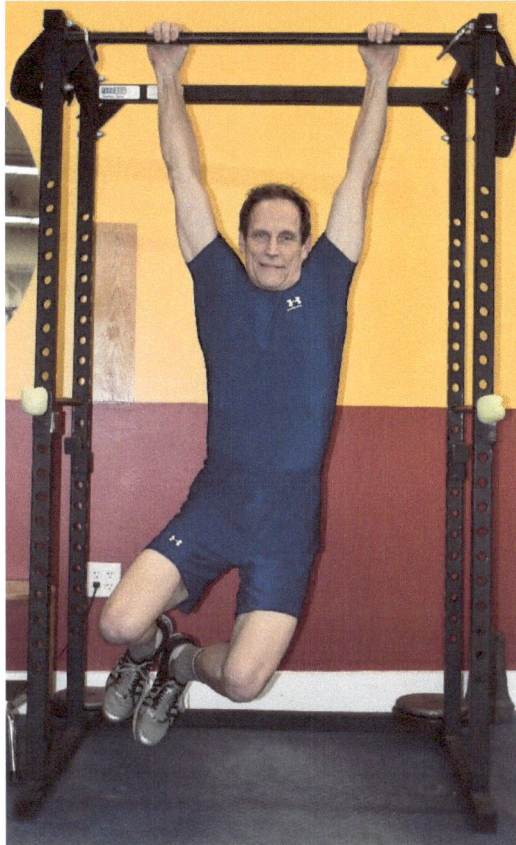

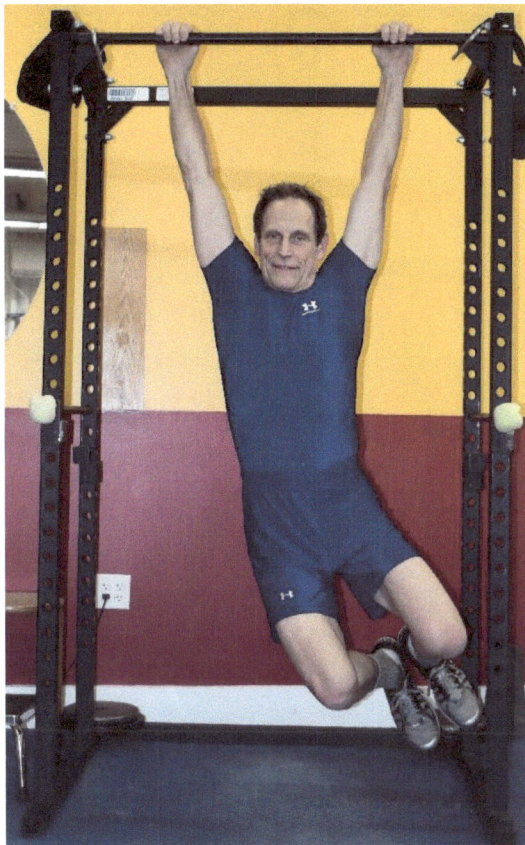

5. Hanging Lower Torso Twist

a. Target Muscles: External and Internal Obliques; Rotational Muscles of the Lower Spine and Hips.

b. As you perform this exercise you will feel mild traction in the lower segments of your spine.

c. Directions

(1) Hang from a bar, bend your knees to 90°, inhale and do abdominal vacuum, the Beginning Position (**Below, this page**).

(2) Exhale, rotate your hips leftward until your target muscles are tightly contracted, pause in the left Peak Position (**Top**).

(3) Inhale, do an abdominal vacuum, and return to the Beginning Position. Pause.

(4) Exhale, rotate your hips rightward until your target muscles are tightly contracted, pause in right Peak Position (**Bottom**). (5) Do 10 repetitions to each side on an alternating basis.

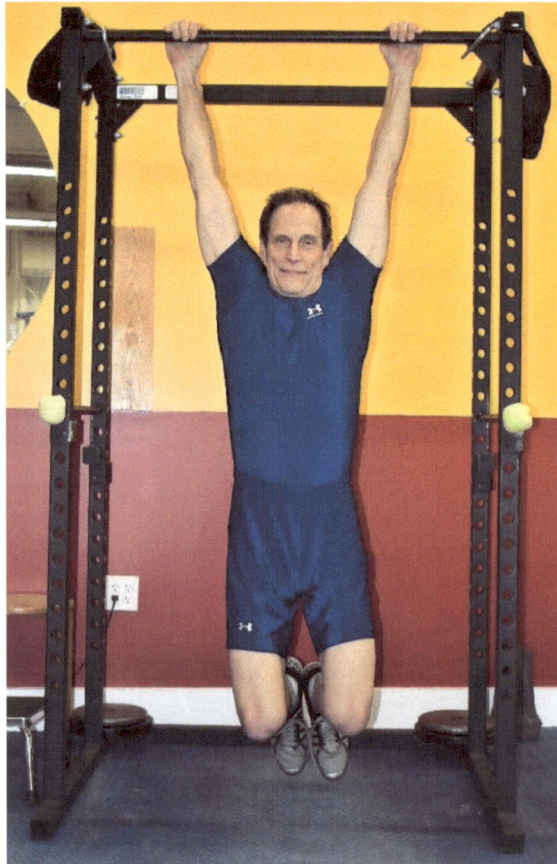

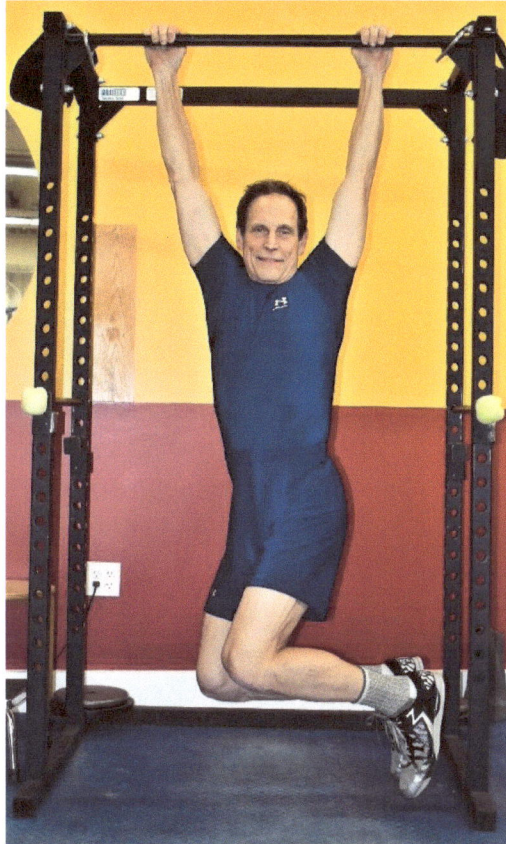

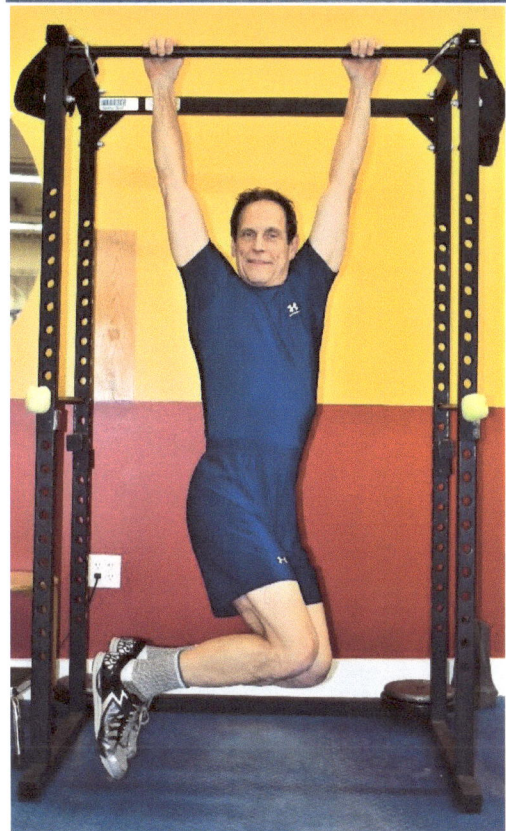

6. Medicine Ball Abdominal Curl on Flat Bench

    a. Target Muscles: Lower and Upper Rectus Abdominis, Transverse Abdominis, Flexors of the neck

    b. By performing this exercise with a 15-20 pound medicine ball, we increase the challenge for our abdominals. By performing it on a bench, we increase significantly the range of motion relative to what we could do on the floor and, at the same time, provide greater stability than doing a similar exercise on an agility ball.

    c. Directions

        1) With a 15-20 pound medicine ball in both hands, recline backward over the length of a weight bench. With your hands overhead and the back of your head just over the end of the bench, allow the ball to descend backward and downward toward the floor, allowing a slight bend in your elbows. This is the Beginning Position (**Top**). You should feel a great stretch in your entire ribcage. Pause, perform an abdominal vacuum, and inhale.

        2) As you begin to exhale, initiate an upward and forward curling motion of your torso by performing a lower abdominal curl. Very smoothly, continue curling your torso and head forward and upward by performing an upper abdominal curl. The **Middle** photo shows the halfway position. Rather than lifting it with your arms, allow the ball to drag behind, keeping maximal stress on your target abdominal muscles.

        3) Continue exhaling as you curl your torso and head upward and toward your feet until the entire length of your abdominal musculature feels fully contracted. This is the Peak Position (**Bottom**). Pause momentarily.

        4) Inhale and perform an abdominal vacuum as your lower your torso and head slowly to Beginning Position. Pause.

        5) As you begin to exhale, use your lower rectus abdominis once again to initiate the next repetition. Enjoy 10-15 exciting repetitions.

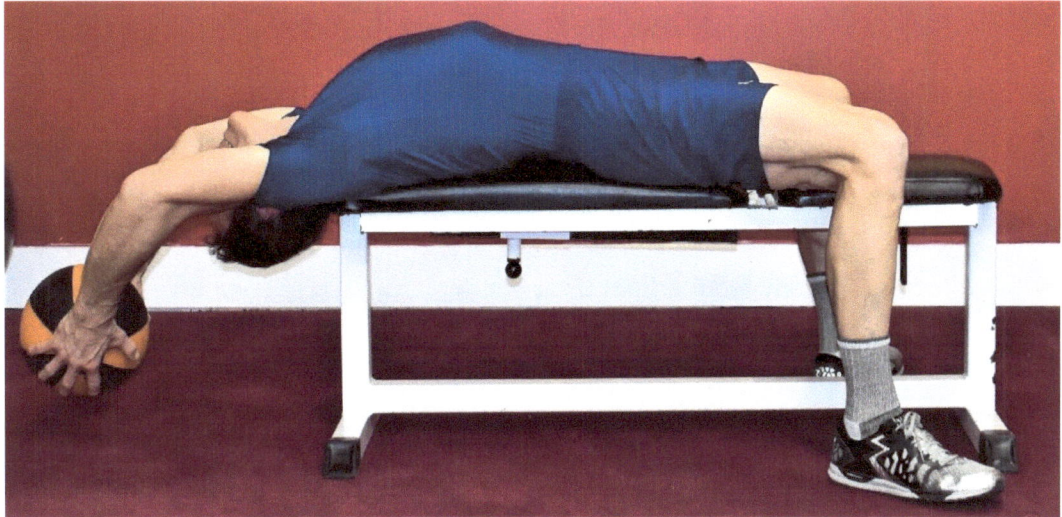
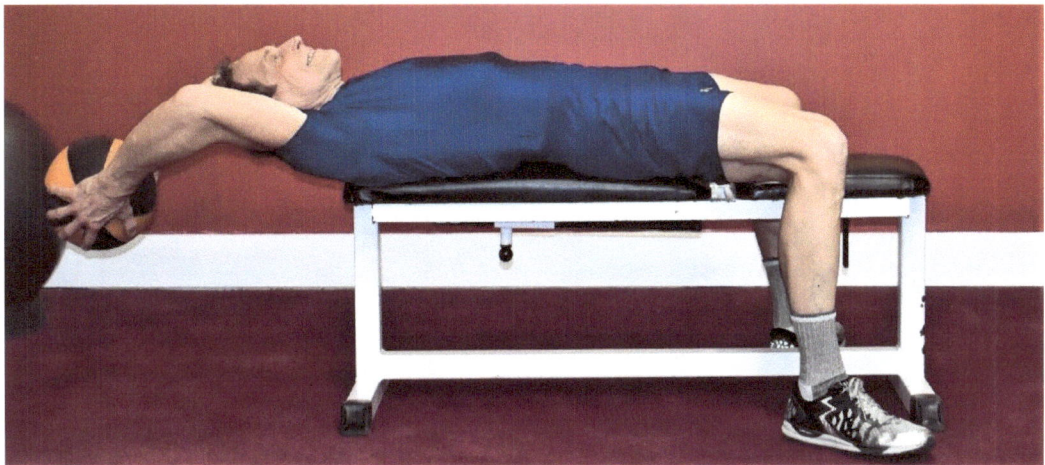
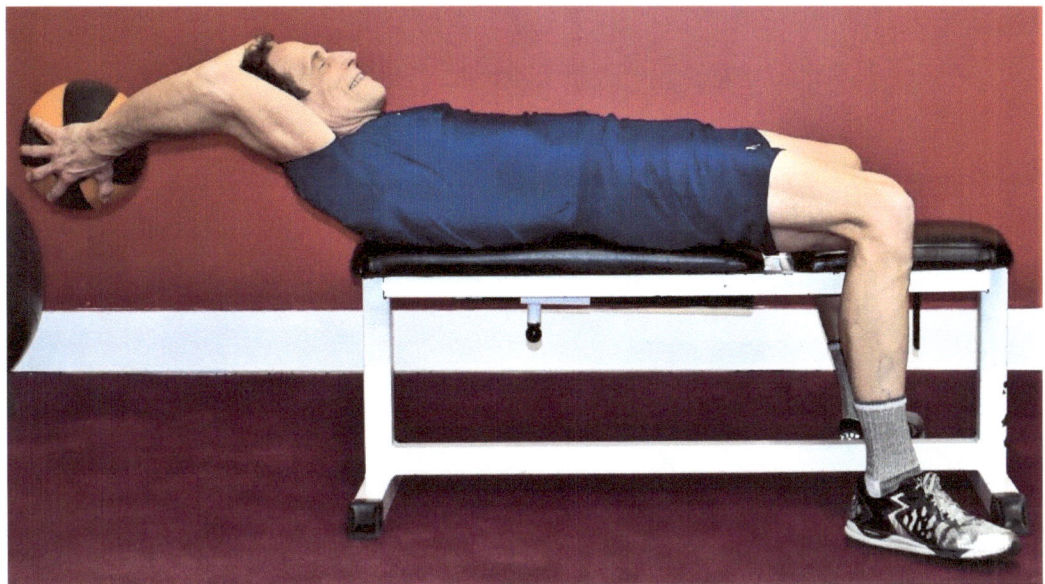

7. Superman: Full Spine Flexion and Extension from the Prone Position

    a. Target Muscles: Extensor muscles of the entire spine, hips, and shoulders.

    b. Very simply, this exercise just feels great!

    c. Directions

        1) Lie face down along the length of a padded weight bench with your head over the top end. With your knees straight and your ankles dorsiflexed, allow your legs to descend toward the floor until you feel a stretch in your hamstrings.

        2) Simultaneously, raise your straightened arms backward and then upward toward the ceiling until you feel a stretch in the front of your shoulders. Inhale in the Beginning Position (**Top**).

        3) As you begin to exhale, slowly lift your head, contract the muscles of your back and hips, and bring your arms downward.
             Middle photo is the halfway position.

        4) Continue to exhale as you raise your head and torso until you are looking straight ahead. Simultaneously, raise your arms straight out in front of you, extend all the muscles of your spine and hips, and point your toes backward.

        5) Pause momentarily in the Peak Position (**Bottom**) to savor the super sensation of whole-body extension.

        6) As you begin to inhale, allow your body to return slowly to the Beginning Position. Enjoy 10 exciting repetitions.

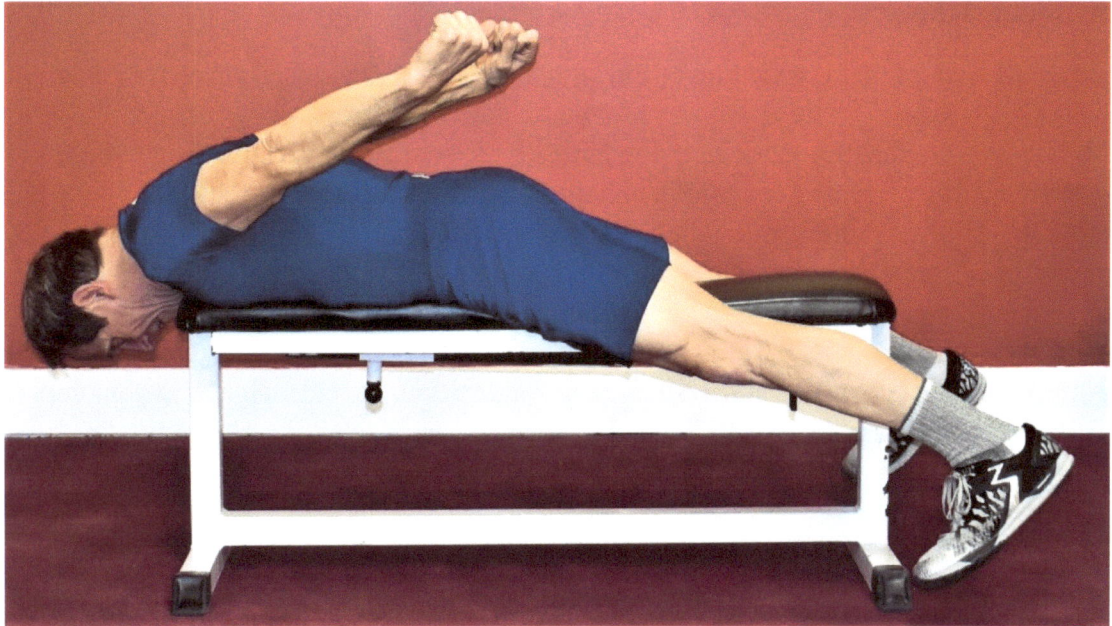

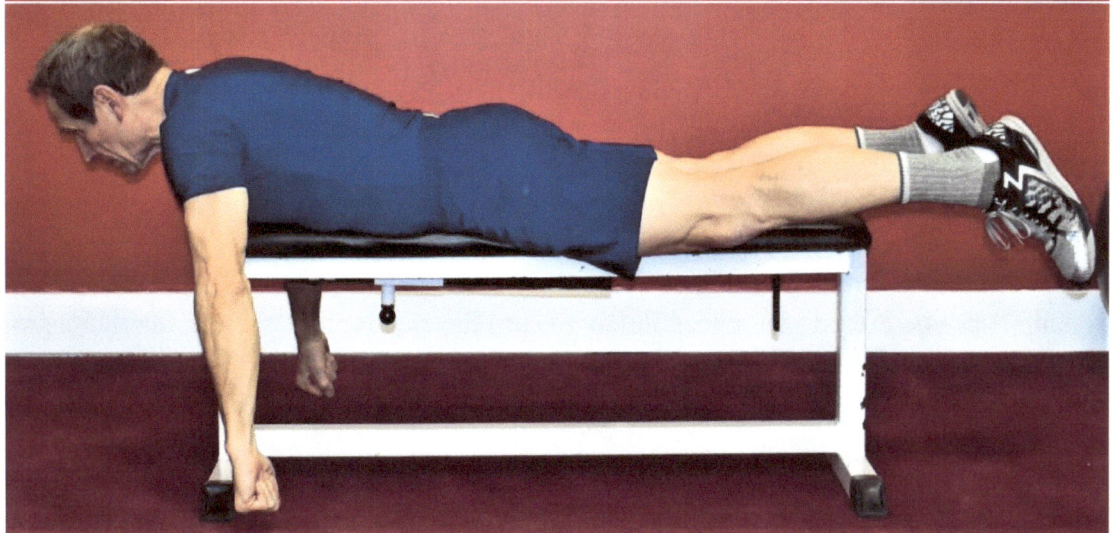

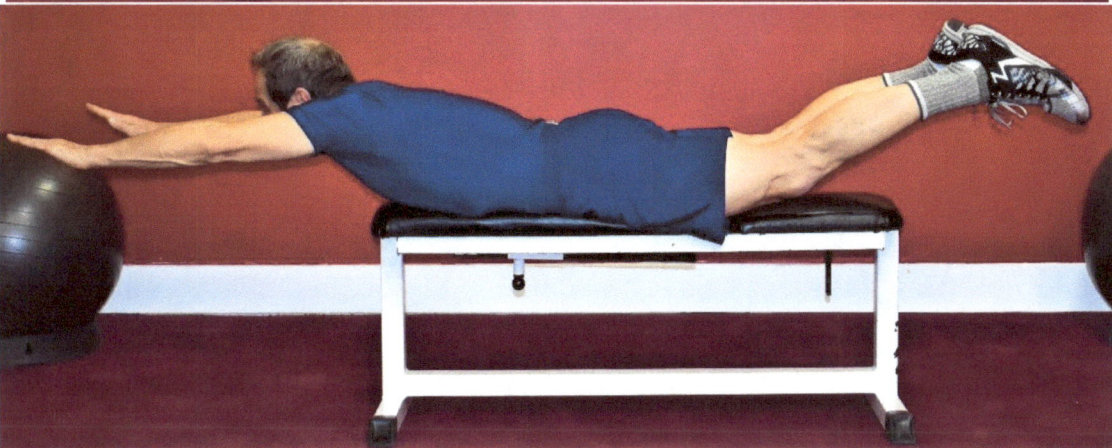

8. Supine Double Knee Raise

a. Target Muscles: Hip Flexors, Lower and Upper Rectus Abdominis, Transverse Abdominis, Neck Flexors

b. Do not even attempt this exercise if you have a history of lower back pain <u>and</u> you have mastered every preceding exercise in volumes 1 and 2 of the Abdominal Strength for Life® program. To every trainee with whom I speak, including myself, I issue the following caveat regarding any exercise: **"When in doubt, leave it out."** No single exercise is worth doing if it increases your risk for injury and, hence, diminishes your health. On the other hand, if you have mastered all the preceding exercises and you are able to do this exercise safely, you will have a profound awareness of how much strength and agility you have developed in your core muscles. This pertains not only to your abdominal and hip flexor muscles, but also to the flexor muscles of your neck. We cannot do advanced abdominal muscles safely or well if the muscles of the neck are weak.

c. Directions

(1) Lie on your back on the floor with your knees straight and arms and hands extended at your sides. Use your neck flexors to curl your head forward slightly. Perform an abdominal vacuum and inhale.

(2) Without moving your legs but keeping your knees straight, exhale and perform a lower abdominal curl, which will push your lower back down against the floor. Photo (**6.69**) is the Beginning Position. Inhale.

(3) As you begin to exhale, perform an upper abdominal curl, flex your head toward your feet, and bend your knees as you draw your feet slowly upward toward your chest. Photo **6.70** is the Peak Position. Pause momentarily to savor an incredibly intense experience.

(4) Inhale as you extend your knees slowly toward the Beginning Position. Maintain strong pelvic tilt, lower abdominal curl, and head flexion positions. Now keep your heels a few inches above the floor as you fully extend your knees. This is the Beginning Position for repetitions 2-10 (**6.71**). Pause momentarily.

(5) Repeat Steps (**3**)-(**4**) for a total of 10 repetitions.

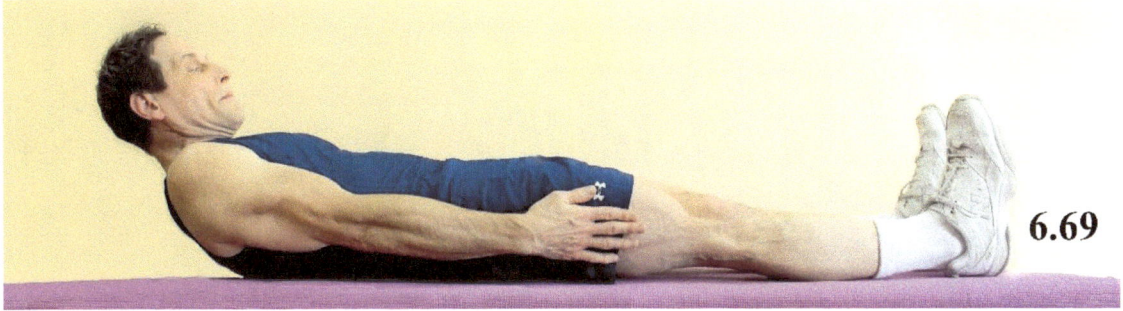

6.69

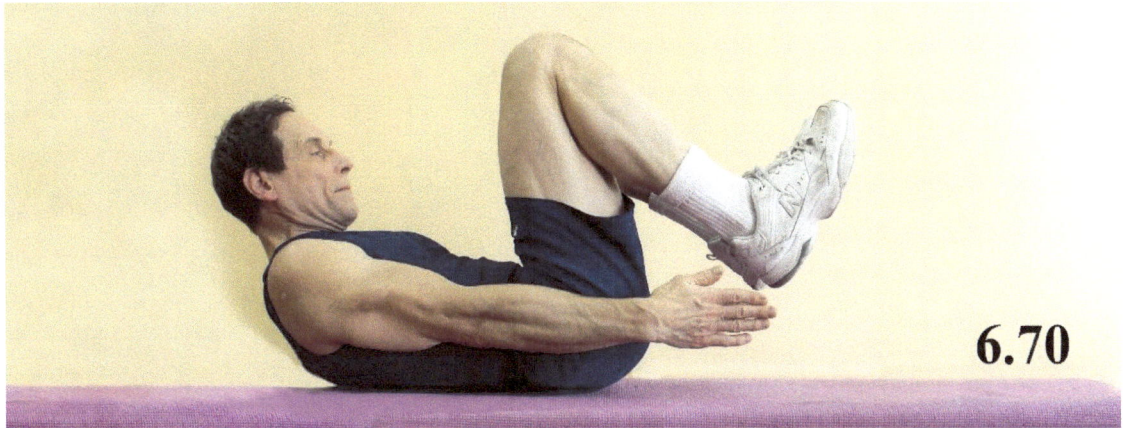

6.70

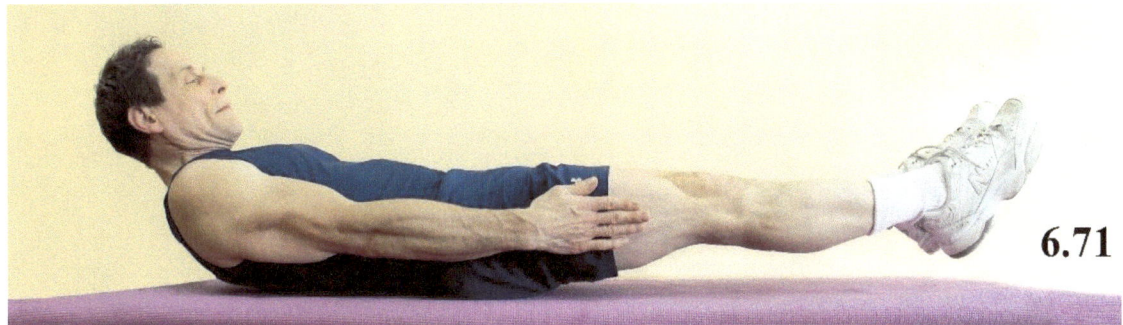

6.71

the Strength for Life® Podcast

With

Dr. Josef Arnould

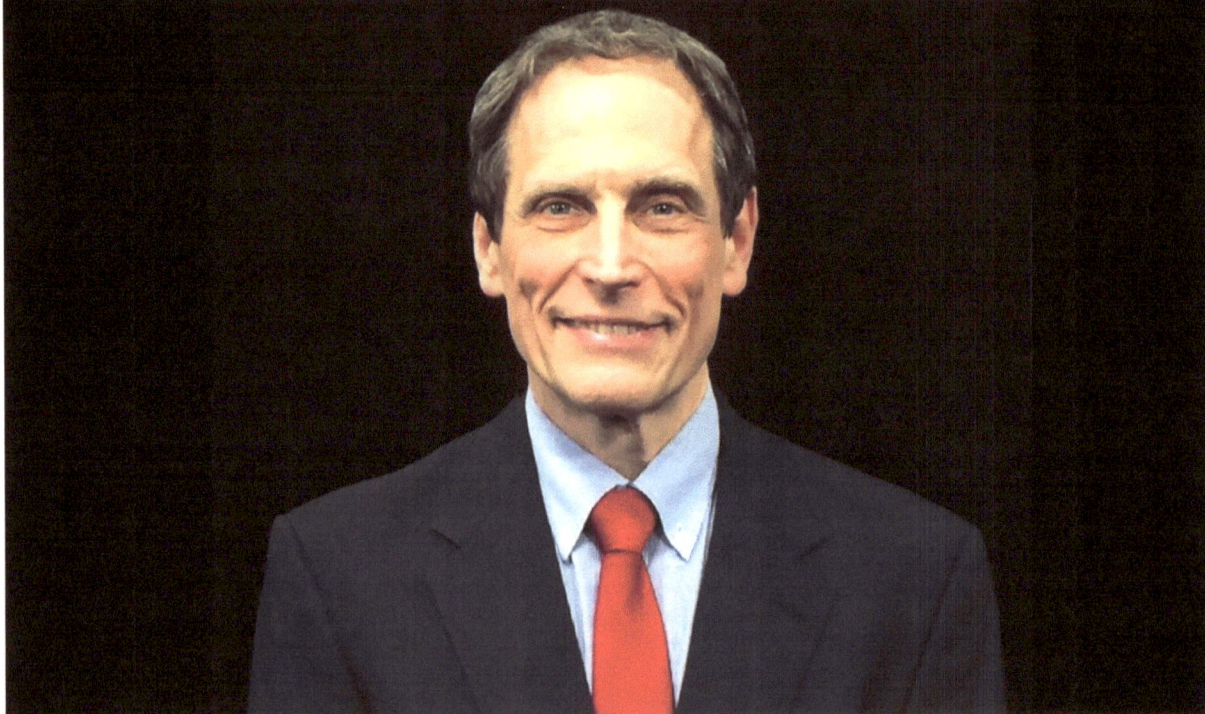

For more than 55 years, I have enjoyed practicing strength training several days each week. In addition, for the past 35 years I have had the privilege of teaching this discipline to people of all ages. During this time, I have also read extensively in the ever-growing field of human nutrition. Based upon these experiences and my ongoing studies in these fields, I feel a great responsibility to share everything I know about the benefits of exercising intelligently and eating nutritiously. Therefore, I cordially invite everyone who has enjoyed reading this book to take advantage of several other learning opportunities available on our clinic website, www.StrengthForLife.com. In addition to Strength for Life® podcasts, as shown above, there are videocasts, blogposts, newsletters, books and e-books, and other educational instruments available for free or at modest costs. I urge you to visit our website and take advantage of these educational opportunities.

Chapter Five

Now That We Have Mastered Core Exercises

Looking Backward

1. First, as I stated at the beginning of this adventure, even the most difficult advanced core exercises are merely complex combinations of the six fundamental exercises that together constitute Medley #1, which begins volume one of this two-part series. This pertains especially to the Lower Abdominal Curl, the first exercise of the entire Abdominal SfL program, and to the Abdominal Vacuum. After appearing initially as separate exercises, they become integrated components of virtually every exercise that follows. Those of us who are able to perform the Supine Double Bent Knee Raise, the last and most difficult exercise of the final advanced core medley, know for certain that it can only be executed safely when we are able to maintain a continuous and powerful lower abdominal curl.

2. Secondly, after mastering these advanced exercises, we know that, to develop flexible strength throughout the entire muscular core, we must perform a wide variety of highly distinct exercises. Simply rattling off hundreds or even thousands of "ab crunches" or "sit-ups" every day (as some people actually do) is woefully inadequate for the development of physical integrity in all the interrelated muscle groups of what we now understand to be and call our "core."

Looking Forward

1. You do <u>not</u> necessarily need to perform every exercise in every medley of this book to reach your goal of attaining a lean, strong, and muscular core. Not every exercise is appropriate for everyone. If one or a few exercises do not feel right to you, eliminate them from your training program. One of our Strength for Life® mantras is: **"When in doubt, leave it out.**

2. You do not necessarily have to organize your core medleys in the same way as they are presented here. Organize your own medleys according to what your experience tells you is effective for you.

3. You do not have to do advanced exercises each day you train your core. Personally, once per week I do only Medley #1 in volume 1, the beginning level workout of this entire program. Similarly, once per week I do each of the two intermediate level workouts, Medleys #2 and #3, of volume 1. Then, once per week I do each of the three advanced medleys presented in this book.

4. You will reach a point in many advanced core exercises where you feel as though you need to perform more than the 10 repetitions recommended in this book. This is natural and can be beneficial. However, be certain you are not misled into thinking you should do 25, 30, or more. Increase the number of repetitions you do in any exercise gradually, by one or two repetitions, **up to a maximum of 20.** Each of the advanced exercises in this book is intensive. If you find yourself feeling as though you need to do more than 20 repetitions, it is very probable you are no longer concentrating as intently as you must to derive the most benefit from every single repetition you perform.

5. Although the medleys of the Abdominal Strength for Life® program are comprised of 42 different exercises, these exercises are not the end all of core muscle training. Not only will you probably leave out a few or several of these from your own training, you will undoubtedly discover other effective exercises that you will want to add to your personal program. This is great! It means you are making your core workouts your own. Congratulations!

6. Once you master the advanced core exercises in this book and practice them regularly, you will be amazed at how much more skilled and proficient you have become in performing the myriad of other physical activities you choose to enjoy in your life.

The Senior Games

A day or two after my 68th birthday, I took a stroll through the athletic field of a local school. I came across a discus ring, an eight-foot circular cement slab surrounded on three sides by tall steel poles and netting. For a wistful moment, I felt regret that in my youth I had only participated in the major "ball" sports. I wished I had tried to throw the discus or participated in one of the other track and field events that are televised during the Olympic Games every four years. I thought, "I might have been able to do pretty well in some of those events or at least had a lot of fun trying."

A few minutes later, as I continued my walk, I recalled reading an article in our local newspaper the previous year. The article described how a 94-year-old man from our community had won the 100-meter dash for his age group in something called the Massachusetts Senior Games. A light bulb switched on in my brain. I thought, "If someone 26 years older than me can participate in track and field events, why can't I try something like that." I walked back to the discus ring, looked at it carefully and at the chalk lines leading away from it that formed a pie-shaped wedge in the field beyond. I said to myself, "Yeah, I can do that." As I walked back home, I thought, "I'm all in" and, "I think this is going to be fun."

Within a few days, I had looked up "Senior Games" on my computer and discovered they were held not just in Massachusetts, but in every state in the U.S. I signed up to participate in the nearby Connecticut Senior Games because their website was open for registration while that for my state was not yet ready to accept registrations. I ordered a book on how to perform Olympic throwing events as well the recommended types of shoes and practice equipment.

My first few training sessions were a strong lesson in humility. While I had dreamed of the discus soaring high and far, as in the pictures in the book and in videos online, I could barely get the thing to "fly" 30 or 40 feet. Nevertheless, it was fun trying. I knew right away I was hooked. Week by week I practiced as much as I able to fit into my work schedule. My form and distances improved little by little, not as much as I would have hoped, but at least enough to keep me motivated.

Approximately eight weeks later, on a Saturday in the middle of May, I drove to New Britain, Connecticut to participate in my first Senior Games. I arrived early, about 7:30 a.m., so I could scope out the site and get a feel for things. As I approached the registration table, I was astonished to see dozens of my fellow and sister "competitors," by appearances in their 50s to 90s, who were already warming up and getting ready for the competition. Very soon, I was even more astonished by the friendly, outgoing, and gracious nature of everyone I met. Most people did not wait for me to address them; they extended a hand, said hello, introduced themselves, and asked for my name and where I was from. I knew instantly that I was in the company of a very special group of people. It was truly an uplifting human experience

After the women's competition at the discus venue was completed, I lined up with my fellow participants for the men's discus. We were separated into 5-year age groups, my classification being for ages 65 to 69, which included about a dozen athletes. We all took a few practice throws, during which there was a lot of friendly banter, and then four throws each in the real competition. I was stunned by how supportive and inspirational nearly every participant was toward his fellow competitors. A few hours before, none of these athletes knew who I was. Now they were encouraging me to do my best. It was a powerful expression of good sportsmanship, precisely what I had learned in Boy Scouts and in Little League.

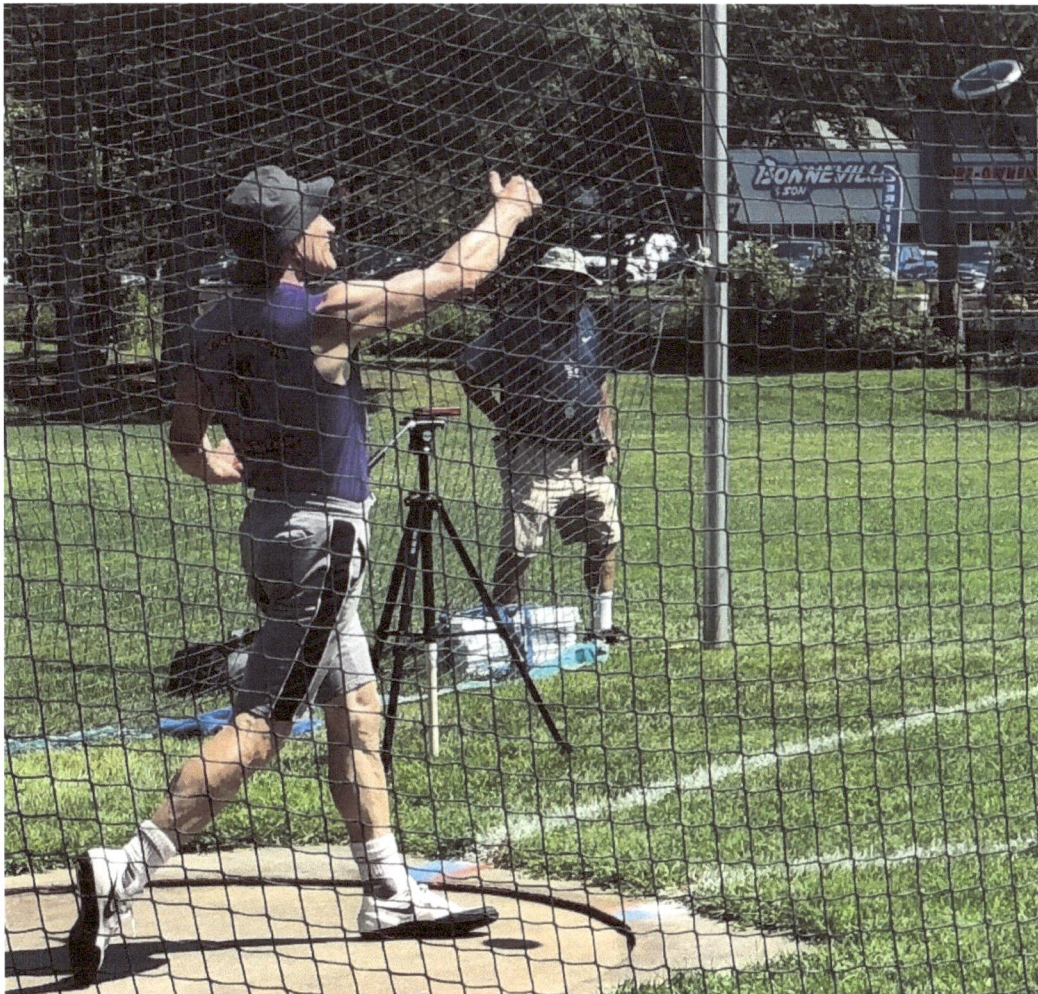

Did I win a gold medal in those games? No, I think I finished 5th or 6th in my age division. But who the heck cared? The good will and outgoing friendliness I had experienced and felt while participating in the Connecticut Senior Games that Saturday far exceeded whatever elation I would have felt if I had thrown the discus 150 feet and won a medal.

Over the past four years, I have continued to practice the discus and, whenever my schedule permits, to participate in the Senior Games of the various New England states. Each year my technique has improved a little bit and the distances of my throws have crept upward, which is personally gratifying. But much more gratifying are the interpersonal relationships I have developed with my fellow and sister participants. This confirms something I have always suspected: there is great joy in being physically active well into the advanced decades of human life. I believe it is this joy that Senior Games athletes enjoy sharing so generously with each other.

Why do I describe all this? I hope to encourage each of you to learn about the Senior Games in your state. Even if you think now that you would not want to participate yourself, you will get a kick out of just going to your local games and watching your fellow and sister superaged adults express themselves in vigorous physical activities.

To learn the date and location of the Senior Games in your state, simply type into your web browser the name of your state followed by "Senior Games." Some states call their games "Master's Games" or "Olympic Games," but "Senior Games" will get you to the website for your state.

The Senior Games are truly inspirational affairs. They remind us to not dwell on physical activities we are no longer able to do, but instead, to search for new and invigorating physical challenges we can enjoy. They remind us also that we must strive constantly to cultivate the quality of health we call strength. Finally, the Senior Games remind us that, to reach our individual potentials for good health and physical independence, each of us must continue exercising vigorously for as long in life as possible.

Josef Arnould, D.C.

DrJosef@StrengthForLife.com

www.ingramcontent.com/pod-product-compliance
Lightning Source LLC
Chambersburg PA
CBHW060900270326
41935CB00004B/53